WATERWORKS

WATERWORKS
Water Therapies for Health and Fitness

D. Baloti Lawrence

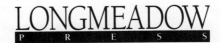

LONGMEADOW
P R E S S

Published by Longmeadow Press, 201 High Ridge Road,
Stamford, CT 06904. No part of this book may be produced or
used in any form or by any means, electronic or mechanical,
including photocopying, recording, or by any information
storage and retrieval system, without permission in writing
from the publisher.

Library of Congress Cataloging-in-Publication Data

Lawrence, D. Baloti

Waterworks: water therapies for health and fitness/D. Baloti
Lawrence: [photos by Phillip Collins; illustrations by Fred Bush].

p.   cm.
1.   Hydrotherapy-Popular words.   I. Title.
RM811.L38   1989   89-8418 CIP
615.8′53-dc20

ISBN: 0-681-41410-3

Printed in the United States of America
1   2   3   4   5   6   7   8   9   10

While preparing this, my fourth book, it was my pleasure to
receive guidance, assistance, or inspiration from the following
individuals: Adrienne Ingrum, who has provided editorial
expertise for each of my books for nearly a decade;
Joan Winokur, who has provided administrative assistance;
Ann Dix, whose sharp skills saved me hours of typing;
and Phillip Collins, for his sensitive camera.
In addition, thank you Lanessa Terry, Marguerite Wong,
Rosie Haas, Dina McDonald, and Karen Lawrence.

At the heart of all things in this world is a place that from the beginning of the universe has been unchanging in one absolute factor. In fact, it may be the only absolute that we know.

At the core of this world, everything is one, everything is equal and everything can be in complete harmony. Everywhere we are the same, one heart, one life, one pulse. At the root of everything there is but one nature, one element and one being.

—DBL, 1989

Contents

1. WATER   9
2. WATER AS HEALER   21
3. THERAPEUTIC BATHS   35
4. WHIRLPOOL BATHS AND HOT TUBS   77
5. SPRINKLE, SPRINKLE:
   THE BENEFITS OF A SHOWER   81
6. SAUNAS   95
7. STEAM BATHS   103
8. ENEMAS AND COLONICS   107
9. COMPRESSES AND PACKS   111
10. ICE: A REMEDY FOR ACHES AND PAINS   123
11. HOT SPRINGS AND NATURAL SPAS   129
12. HOW TO FIX IT WITH WATER   137
13. DRINKING WATER   147
14. A WET FUTURE   151

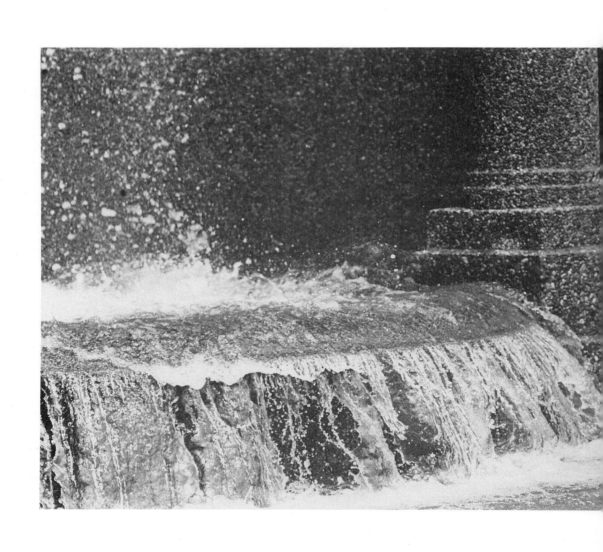

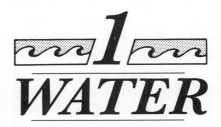

WATER

The qualities of water go far beyond the typical bath, or even its use as a sparkling beverage. In folklore, water is closely associated with the essence of all life on earth. It represents deep inner awareness, flowing movement, intuition and subtle power. Water is, in fact, the best representation we have for the origin of life. It is said that the anatomy and physiology of humans resemble those of animals and plants. All three contain many of the same elements found in the oceans. Just as the greatest percentage of the human body is made up of water, so the earth's surface is primarily water. Water is everywhere. Water is in everything. Where there is no water, there is no life. There is a subtle energy in water formed by the union of its hydrogen and oxygen molecules. The partnership of two of nature's most incredible elements gives water a flexibility and durability that serve many purposes in our lives.

From sports to health and beauty, this vibrant natural element lives, breathes, expands, contracts and moves through our environment, touching almost every phase of our lives. It is subtle but strong, mutable but stable, passive yet indestructible.

There is an interplay between all living things on this earth. Look at this simple example: a rain cloud will eventually wet the soil, which will, in turn, feed the plants, which then produce food, which ultimately feeds us. Because water is the source of fluid for all the world, it affects every event in the life process. To call water simply a vital substance is an understatement—it is healthful, it is fun, it is beautifying . . . it is water!

Water is thus the universal element. This book introduces the techniques available to us, and what we need to know, to use water for its maximum benefits.

For years, I have known about—and used—many marvelous water treatments. While some techniques were previously available only at special health spas or resorts, many now can be brought into your home. This book simplifies them for easy practical use. It provides step-by-step information on water techniques and therapies that will improve your health, help relieve your aches and pains and enhance your physical beauty.

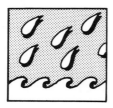 *H_2O*

In 1785, Antoine Lavoisier proved that water is composed of two parts of hydrogen and one part of oxygen. The symbol for water is thus given as H_2O. Water in a pure state is a transparent, odorless, tasteless liquid.

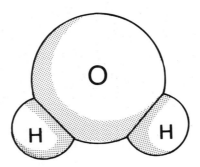

The water molecule has a peculiar pyramid-shaped structure that gives it properties unlike any other molecule.

Characteristics of Water

Freezes at .32°F or 0°C and boils at 212°F or 100°C.

Contains 11.188% hydrogen and 88.812% oxygen by weight.

Comes in three forms: liquid, solid and gas, of which there are many variations—snow, spring, sweet, cold, hot, tepid, fresh, hard, soft.

The most abundant chemical on earth.

Makes up approximately 70% of the human body.

Has tremendous solvent action; more substances will dissolve in it than in any other liquid.

Usually makes up 20–90% of all animal and plant tissue.

Can be heated to 2000°C without appreciable decomposition.

Has magnetic and electric power.

Contains minerals that nourish the body.

Water moves in a continuous circle on a journey from the earth to the atmosphere, and back again to earth. While 75% of the earth is covered with water of some type, water changes form frequently. A great deal of water is captured in glaciers, while other water is trapped in clouds and still other water creates the depth of oceans and seas. Water created billions of years ago may still exist. The water in your home may have existed for tens of thousands of years in the glacier that covers Greenland until sunlight set it free to join the clouds, only to fall to earth again.

It has been said that water is the Eighth Wonder. Many tests have concluded that its potency is due in great part to its unique structure. When the two parts of hydrogen and the one part of oxygen come together, they form the compound known as water. Both hydrogen and oxygen are valuable elements in their own right. Hydrogen, the most common element, constitutes some 90% of all the matter in the universe. It is the element of outer space, since most of the free hydrogen rises. Lower levels of the atmosphere have practically no free hydrogen. Oxygen is the second most abundant element on the planet. It is the element of combustion. It is the eager joiner, the stirrer-up of elements. In fact, it is a 20% component of the air we breathe. Its molecular structure gives water its remarkable powers. It has the simplicity of form of the pyramids. It can draw in, hold and carry in its essence all sorts of ions, atoms and molecules of other elements without impairing itself.

The instant hydrogen touches free oxygen in the air, the two elements dart together by electrostatic magnetism. The result is water. This process still occurs wherever volcanic activity is releasing hydrogen gas from rocks deep in the earth's crust. New water is visible as steam when water vapor is cooled in the air. It is the eerie mist that hovers over a volcanic mountain. A spectacular sight is the vision of water forming in the Alaskan valleys or the Hawaiian mountains where steam is still rising as the vapor cools. Often the hissing of sparkling mist can be heard as new water molecules are born. As the sun is mostly hydrogen, this element brings its fiery, energizing qualities to water. No wonder water is such a vibrant element!

Pure water is virtually unknown, as almost all water has some mineral or chemical contents. Carbonic acid, a mixture of water and carbon dioxide, falls to the earth through rain, and according to scientists has a special vitalizing effect on our water bodies.

Hard and Soft Water

There are two basic kinds of water: hard and soft. Soft water lathers readily with soap. Hard water does not dissolve it as easily, because it already contains dissolved minerals. Rainwater is soft water; it does not contain much calcium or magnesium. The hardness or softness of water can be temporary or permanent. Permanent hard water contains dissolved calcium or magnesium sulfate and cannot be softened by boiling. It must be treated with chemicals that will remove the calcium or magnesium. Temporary hard water contains dissolved calcium or magnesium bicarbonate and can be softened by boiling, as well as by the addition of lime. Both types can be softened by passing them through modern water softeners. You can very often see the chemical residues left in bottles, pipes or tea kettles.

Fresh Water

Although water looks clear, there are many things dissolved in it. When materials are dissolved in water, it becomes a solution. Drinking water is a solution. Although it looks pure, there are gases, minerals and other substances in it. When rain falls, water molecules dissolve gases in the air; when a river or stream passes over rocks or soil, or seeps through them, the water dissolves minerals and salts from the rocks and soil. Flowing water will also dissolve material such as pesticides or other toxins in the soil. In fact, water will dissolve anything it touches to some degree. Some minerals in water have a beneficial effect on us, while others can be harmful.

Fresh water is found in springs, rivers and some inland sources. Fresh water does not taste salty, and the taste may vary, depending on the source from which it came. Fresh waters will have a different chemical balance and a different taste when they come from different springs. An urgent question regarding the future is how to prevent the destruction of fresh-water sources and how to get fresh water from sea water at a reasonable cost.

Salt Water

Ocean or salt water is unsuitable for human consumption, although it may possess rejuvenating qualities for the skin and muscles. In large quantities, it is toxic to the human body. Salt water is equally unsuitable for plant growth. Three-fourths of the water in the ocean contains common table salt, sodium chloride. In addition, the potency of this water is enhanced by the fifty or so different elements found in natural sea water. The sea yields precious minerals that we extract and use, from gold to diamonds to uranium, not to mention oil.

The U.S. Government has set up a plant where sea water is converted into fresh water. The greatest cost in the conversion involves the fuel needed to run the stills. After adding the salaries of employees, the cost of equipment and maintenance, it is clear that desalinization is not now cost-effective.

Let tap water run at full force for two or three minutes the first thing in the morning. This will help clean out high levels of lead and copper that may have built up overnight in the pipes.

Water Purification Methods

Regular tap water can be made fresh by several purification methods.

Filtration is the passing of natural water through beds of sand and gravel to hold back suspended matter and most of the bacteria, and sometimes also through charcoal filters to remove odorous gases, such as ammonia.

Aeration is the spraying of water into the air. This helps to oxidize the organic matter, as well as to remove objectionable odors and tastes.

Chlorination is the addition of chlorine to water to destroy bacteria.

Distillation involves the vaporization of water, followed by condensation to remove all of the volatile solids. Distilled water is the purest form of water available.

Boiling heats water to its point of agitation, which occurs at 212°F. It can have a minimal benefit for purification. It does not remove any solid material, but does kill bacteria.

For more information on drinking water and water purity, refer to Chapter 13.

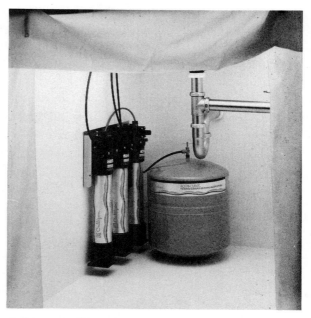

An under-the-sink water filtration device.
Photo courtesy of Culligan of Connecticut.

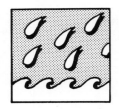

WATER IN ANCIENT HISTORY

In 3200 B.C., the first recorded evidence of a public water system existed. Some years later, King Menes of Egypt dammed the Nile River and manipulated its course to better serve his country's need for water. Records also show the existence of the Indus Valley water supply department in India. There were vast water departments in China and South America as well, and later throughout Europe. The oldest dam in the world is said to be the Gardwii, about 18 miles south of Cairo, Egypt. In ancient Egypt, the *Wafa* was the day of celebration and fasting, when dikes were cut to allow the life-giving water to flood the land. This was both mentally and physically rewarding for the populace, as they hoped during this time for a good crop in the upcoming season.

It was not long before humans found out about the rejuvenating and beautifying benefits of water. Maidens were known to soak in baths of natural spring water. To this water were often added special oils or exotic flowers. The benefits of the beauty bath ranged from soothing tired muscles to creating a velvety soft skin. Special flowers such as roses, jasmine or lilies were picked at special times and stored in airtight jars. When the flowers were dried, they were then crushed and added to boiling water to extract their essence.

In still another process, precious oils were extracted from aromatic herbs and flowers and mixed with palm or coconut oil. Trained attendants then massaged bathers using the oils after they had been mildly warmed. In addition, linen or cotton cloths were soaked in the warm oil and then applied to certain parts of the body for their soothing effect.

Ancient saunas consisted of small wooden structures (much resembling today's saunas) within which heated coals trapped heat, which then created steam. Aromatic and fragrant oils were placed in the saunas to add a pleasant atmosphere.

Known for their tremendous healing properties, natural bodies of water such as the Nile, the Euphrates, the Black Sea and the Mediterranean Sea were visited by thousands who soaked in their waters, believing them to produce everything from fertility and relief from aches and pains to purification of the soul and spiritual well-being.

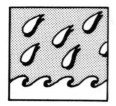

YOUR INNER JUICES

Water is everywhere in the body. In fact, our bodies are approximately 70% to 75% liquid. Without water, our bodies would dehydrate, overheat and shut down completely. Water serves many vital functions:

- facilitates the process of digestion
- transports food to the tissues
- eliminates body toxins
- provides circulation of body fluids
- maintains balance and harmony in the body
- regulates body temperature
- acts as a catalyst to most chemical functions
- helps nourish and feed the body
- helps maintain pH balance
- provides fluid for cells
- helps lubricate and cushion joints

Since water is the ultimate harmonizer, it has the role of regulating and maintaining body balance. The balance between intake and output of water keeps the composition of the body's fluid constant. The intake of water is regulated mostly by the sensation of thirst.

The body does not have a built-in water tank that it can tap into conveniently when it is running dry. Since water is essential for every process in the body, a lack of it leads to mental and physical changes, including prematurely aging skin and muscular weakness.

Drinking too much water is called water intoxication and can be as bad as having too little water. If the body takes in too much water, it is equipped with special cells that will alert it. Heavy perspiration occurs,

Signs of H$_2$O Deficiency

Thirst

Dry mouth

Headache

Nausea

Weakness

Chills

Dry skin or hair

Excessive (or lack of) perspiration

or, as in the prolonged use of diuretics, water is eliminated through frequent urination. Carried from the body in this fluid loss are also valuable minerals and nutrients.

The human embryo is at least 97% water, and in a 150-pound man there are approximately 42 quarts of water. Water is the basic component of all cells. It moves back and forth between the skin, organs, tissues and finally into cells. This bodily process is called osmosis. It keeps the balance in the body. Thus, each of us should drink a minimum of six glasses of water daily. If we perform difficult activities, such as sports or hard work, it is necessary to drink more.

The body has two kidneys. They act as filters that clean the body by removing waste products through the production of urine. This cleaning fluid is, in fact, the flow of impurities leaving our systems.

By drinking water we help the body clean itself both inside and out. As we discharge from our bodies through the kidneys, then the bladder, water acts as the main carrier for toxins to be eliminated from the body. The kidneys separate toxins from usable nutrients.

As salt causes water to be retained in the tissues, excessive salt intake will severely inhibit kidney function and ultimately cause kidney damage. It should be noted that almost all fresh foods contain sodium (salt), while most adulterated or processed foods contain harmful additives and usually extra salt. The average "full diet" usually contains far more salt than necessary. This also leads to high blood pressure, obesity and arthritis. No wonder that when treating any of these, the doctor's first orders are "no more salt."

To keep kidney function healthy, drink plenty of pure water, reduce salt intake and include enough unadulterated foods in your diet.

Drinking sufficient water helps cleanse and filter the all-important blood circulation, giving rise to a healthier and more beautiful skin tone. Water is absolutely essential as a powerful body cleanser and purifier.

Salt

A word must be said here about salt as it relates to the body's sodium content. Common table salt is the form of sodium with which we are most familiar. Salt is necessary to help our kidneys regulate body water and minerals. It also helps to move carbon dioxide through our bodies and maintain our pH balance. Without salt, our kidneys will not function. However, too much salt is unhealthy, because it causes the body to retain water, which will eventually clog up the organs. Sodium stimulates nerve and muscle tissues so they can move. Today, however, because processed foods almost always contain too much salt, most people suffer from too much salt in their bodies rather than too little. Too much salt has been linked directly to hypertension and overweight.

Water is released from the body in several forms. It passes from our eyes as tears, from our skin as perspiration and from cuts as blood. Nursing mothers excrete mostly water in their milk. Our lungs expel water as we exhale.

Perspiration is an important factor in keeping our bodies healthy and fit. It helps the body dispose of excess heat and maintain a normal body temperature. If the body does not have enough water to produce sweat, the body temperature rises to dangerous levels. In addition, with insufficient water, the body's blood volume is reduced, providing less blood to carry oxygen and food nutrients to all parts of the body. As a result of this dehydration, muscles become weak and a feeling of fatigue sets in.

Water is a natural healer for the body. It replenishes and cleanses. A steady amount of fresh water helps keep the skin and pores clean and open, breathing properly for a beautiful, healthy glow.

Another important function that involves water is regulation of the pH (acid-alkaline) balance. The pH balance is important because it represents the difference between an unhealthy body or a fit and active one.

When the pH balance is below 7.4, a state of acidosis occurs; the body is more acid than alkaline. Out of balance in the other direction, a pH above 7.4 produces an alkaline system. Along with our lungs and kidneys, water works to help keep this delicate balance.

Human body temperature should be at 98.6°F for optimal health. Water helps keep this balance as it flows through the body, cooling or heating as needed.

Water helps carry nutrients through the body: Our digestive juices are 99% water and are needed to help our bodies extract nutrients from the foods we eat.

Water is responsible for the growth and function of every cell in the body. And, as if there were not enough uses for water in the body, it also plays an important role in preventing mental burnout: Water is responsible for transmitting messages from cell to cell, in constant communication with the brain.

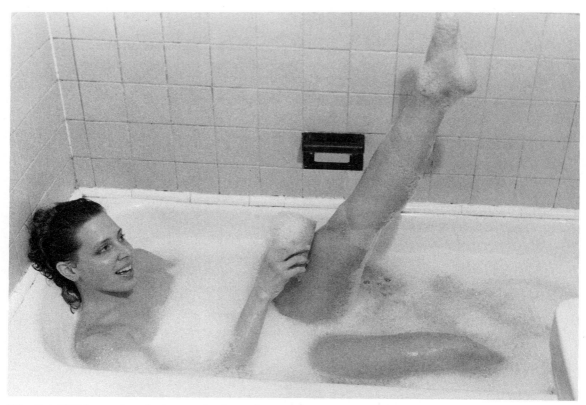

The leg lift is a stimulating technique for toning cellulite and firming stomach muscles. This is one of the many exercises you can do while taking a relaxing bath. Enjoy . . .

2
WATER AS HEALER

Water has the power to aid in the rejuvenation and fitness of our bodies.

In the 19th century, an English physician made this statement about water:

> It does not deal with mere symptoms. It goes at once to the root of the matter. It deals with principles and causes. It does not tinker with the human body and mend it up with patches. It takes a great and general and comprehensive view of ill health and its causes. It claims to be sensible, rational and in harmony with the known laws which regulate and govern life, health, and pleasure. I have shown that the pores of the skin, if joined end to end, would form a tube 28 miles long. Surely, there can be no difficulty in believing that if this tube be obstructed, and the matters which it is intended to carry out of the blood be left in it, while the matters which it is intended to convey into the blood be kept out of it—surely, I say, there can't be difficulty in believing that a very unhealthy and wrong state of blood must be the necessary result. And it must surely be apparent that any treatment which has the power of restoring or augmenting the function of this stupendous secreting tube must be capable of exercising a beneficial influence on health and, through this means alone, of airing many forms of ill health. How plain and commonsense this appears. How rational! How intelligible!

In a recent project, subjects were immersed in cold baths to study the healthful benefits. They were immersed for two hours in chest-deep water. The results were as follows:

- reduction in edema (swollen tissues, often caused by water retention)
- increase in urine flow
- release of excess salt
- 5% decline in blood toxins
- 50% temporary increase in heart function
- one-half kilogram loss in weight
- rise in peripheral blood flow and circulation

Vincent Preissnitz is a name synonymous with the healthy applications of water. He was a farmer who laid the foundation for the modern-day system we call hydrotherapy. Suffering from paralysis in one hand because of an accident, he experimented with water therapy to relieve his hand condition after he was told there was nothing that could be done. He was successful and soon found other applications, as others began to seek him out for his special water cures.

Sebastian Kneipp, born in Bavaria in 1921, was another well-known subscriber to the healing powers of water. He helped to perfect some of Preissnitz's techniques and is also responsible for what is known today as the Kneipp methods.

The best thing about hydrotherapy is that it usually is as pleasurable as it is healthy. It feels *good* while it heals you.

As we travel through the world of water, I will attempt to share information that will help you use this wonderful element. (For example, fitness buffs will discover that weak muscle response may be caused by minor water dehydration, and learn to avoid this by drinking small amounts of neutral spring water during workouts.)

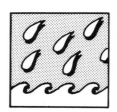

FORMS OF WATER & THEIR BENEFITS

Several forms of water are used when treating or caring for the body:

liquid - water

gas - steam

solid - ice

Hot water can be used internally and externally. It increases blood circulation, increases the movement of everything it comes in contact with and quiets and soothes. Hot compresses are effective for healing and preventing premature aging.

Steam increases cell renewal of the skin, while it offers a natural method for deep cleansing, opening pores and cellular regeneration. Steam relaxes and energizes the body; as it creates perspiration, it cleanses the body from within.

Neutral or tepid water offers an organizer to help balance and regulate all body functions. It is the master harmonizer, as it both cools and warms during its flow through the body.

Hot and cold alternating water applications are by far the best. Changing the temperature between hot and cold offers the body a revitalizing balancing experience.

Hydrotherapy is water in its different forms applied to every part of our existence: mental, physical, spiritual.

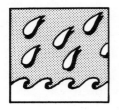

HOW WATER ACTS ON THE BODY

The magical properties of water assist the body in many healing ways:

Restorative tonic—through cold water, whirlpool, coldsprays, packs and hot and cold showers, water stimulates healing action and increases circulation, energizing the total body.

Relaxant—hot and cold compresses, ice bags, warm baths, hot packs, enemas and whirlpool all help to soothe and comfort the body.

Reduce fever—short cold baths, sponging, cold-mitten massage and damp sheet packs help regulate body temperature to lower fevers.

Diuretic—hot packs and drinking water can affect kidney action and help maintain pH balance.

Rubefacient—alternating hot and cold applications of all kinds will increase surface circulation in most areas.

Eliminative—water dissolves, eliminates and extracts toxins and unwanted materials from the body.

Antiseptic—boiling hot water will usually destroy bacteria, and also cleanses the food we eat and sterilizes our environment.

Stimulant—drinking mineral water and taking hot or cold herbal baths will greatly enhance personal energy.

Anesthetic—ice packs will dull uncomfortable feeling or sensations.

Sedative—warm baths, warm packs and hot herbal teas will help soothe and calm the body, reducing the effects of stress and burnout.

How you apply water to receive its optimal benefits depends entirely on your needs and personal choice. There are several techniques for each use. To receive the benefits of hot water, for example, you may use a hot bath, a hot compress or a hot tub. The same is true for tepid water and cold water. These are the main points to consider:

1. What temperature do you wish the water to be—hot, cold, tepid or hot *and* cold?
2. What kind of pressure do you prefer—heavy massage-type, light spray or alternating sprinkle?
3. What is the most effective form for your specific purpose—local heat, local cold, compress, friction, sponging, baths, steam, shower, hot tub, whirlpool, shampoo, enema, colonic, ice, drinking water or sauna?
4. What is the duration of the process you have chosen—30 seconds, 10 minutes, 1 hour?
5. What material or equipment will you need—ice bag, tub, hot compress?

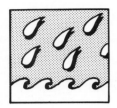

ALL TOGETHER NOW . . .

Water as a therapy is effective alone. However, just like human inter-action, it is best utilized when there is a total approach, a group effort. Water is complemented by and complements so many other elements. Each one may have its own special powers, and when tastefully blended together, all provide greater benefits. The total approach to fitness or health means that the same situation is approached with different tech-niques, each with its own special effect. When using more than one technique, the techniques work like a finely tuned watch, with each el-ement fitting with the others as a part of the whole. For example, some herbal teas can be beneficial in relaxing tense muscles. Therefore, when these herbs are placed in your warm bath water, you have enhanced the benefit to your muscles by 100%. Without listing all of them, I have selected some of the more natural partners of water that are used fre-quently to heal the body.

Nutrition

Good nutrition is a major way of preventing many imbalances in the body. In addition, it is a strong force, able to strengthen, tone and rejuvenate the body. Certain foods, such as refined sugar, white flour products, excessive salt, chemical preservatives, large amounts of red meat, take away from the body's vital energy. They do not contribute to its overall well-being. Instead, fresh fruits, vegetables, whole grains and pure water have rejuvenating and healing properties for the body. It is important that the body receive the proper nutrients to stay fit and healthy. (See page 147 for information on drinking water.)

> When eating, drink a small amount of water before to stimulate the juices. Drink the remainder after eating. Always avoid drinking during your meals for better digestion and assimilation of your food.

Exercise

Some exercise is better than none, and regular exercise is better than some. Exercise and water go hand in hand. There are many water sports and many ways to exercise in water. Exercise helps in the following ways:

- provides aerobic conditioning to increase circulation
- strengthens the body
- increases endurance
- tones muscles for speed and agility
- provides more flexibility
- sharpens mental abilities
- enhances self-esteem
- makes life more enjoyable
- acts as nature's total beauty program

Exercise can provide hours of recreational fun and can be done by anyone. It is necessary to keep the body healthy and fit.

Herbs

Nature has given us plants and flowers that provide good taste, vitamins, minerals and other life-giving essences. Herbs may be used in the form of a compress, pack, infusion, liniment, poultice, tincture, cream, food extract or as a culinary for enhancing taste.

Herbal plants offer at least five parts that are useful in healing preparations: root, stem, leaf, flower and essential oil. While oils may be inhaled or massaged into the skin, leaves and flowers may be taken as teas. Herbal teas can taste quite good—they don't have to taste bad to be good for you!

My Ten Favorite Herbs and Their Uses

PEPPERMINT: If there is one all-around herb to have in your kitchen, it must be effervescent peppermint. In addition to its vitamin and mineral content, this herb tastes delicious when blended with any other herb and is excellent in baths, compresses and tonics.

CAMOMILE: This is the beauty and relaxation herb. Use it to relax after a day's work or when your nerves are frayed. It makes a wonderful beauty aid that softens skin, conditions hair and creates a sweet and aromatic bath.

SAGE: Loaded with natural vitamins, sage makes the perfect hair rinse. Mix it with peppermint for a natural tea. The word means "tea of wisdom," and the herb is reputed to enhance creative thinking.

ROSEMARY: A mild stimulant, rosemary helps to get the body going. Mix it with sage and camomile for the ultimate hair rinse. Rosemary is also very popular with cooks: It serves as a great seasoning in salads and vegetable dishes.

GOLDEN SEAL: Known as a "heal-all," this herb is a good vitamin source for curing colds. It is useful for therapeutic packs, compresses and baths.

KELP: Actually a seaweed, kelp is rich in iodine and B vitamins. When you add it to your bath water, it is like soaking in the ocean.

ROSE HIPS: A great source of Vitamin C, rose hips—mixed well with peppermint—makes a wonderful tea that will help to stave off colds.

DANDELION: Another favorite culinary herb, dandelion is full of vitamins and minerals. Due to its deep roots, which store nourishment from the lower layers of the soil, dandelion makes for a nourishing cup of tea.

LICORICE: Superior for irritated throats, colds and most respiratory problems, licorice is a sweet-tasting herb that can help reduce and eliminate toxins from the body.

ALOE VERA: The perfect herb for soothing cuts and burns, aloe vera should be in every kitchen. Simply break off a piece of the plant and squeeze out its marvelous juice. It is a natural skin moisturizer.

These ten herbs were chosen because of their multi-purpose qualities, availability and practicality. Of course, there are many more to choose from, but these alone should give you hours of health, beauty and culinary delight.

Massage

What better way to relax after a workout than with a relaxing back massage? Massage has both physical and mental benefits. It penetrates deep into tight, tense tissues and gently caresses a nagging headache. In addition, massage communicates well with water. They have total harmony when used together: Massage will help facilitate the use of hydrotherapy, and hydrotherapy will facilitate the use of massage.

Internal energy moves through the body through what are known as energy channels. These channels correspond, in many cases, to the pathways of fluid moving inside the body. Massage can help keep these

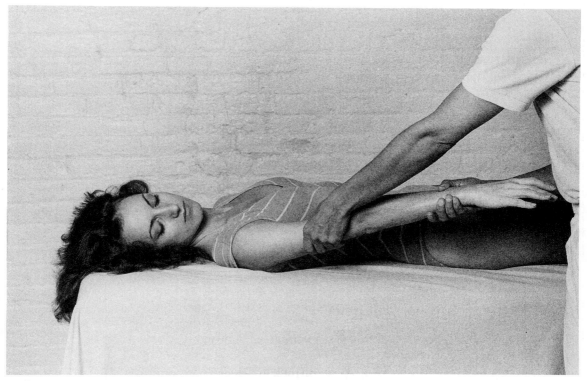

Effleurage: Stroking the arms and hands. Begin at shoulders and use long, firm strokes toward fingertips. Tennis and golf players will appreciate the increase of circulation around a stiff elbow. *Photo by Ebet Roberts*.

channels clear and moving freely. This will result in a higher state of health and well-being.

There are several techniques in massage:

effleurage—long, continuous strokes
percussion—tapping, slapping, chopping movements (always perform gently)
vibration—moving up and down
friction—brisk rubbing or sliding movements
kneading—deep manipulation by fingers as though kneading dough
finger pressure—light to heavy pressure applied by leaning the finger into the massaged area
range of motion—increases movement and activates muscles to prevent weakening and deterioration

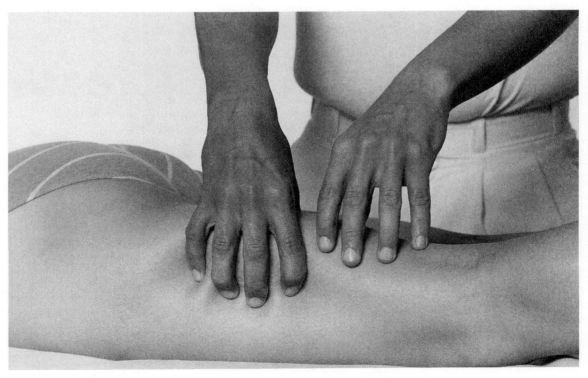

Kneading the thigh. Always work in the direction of the heart.

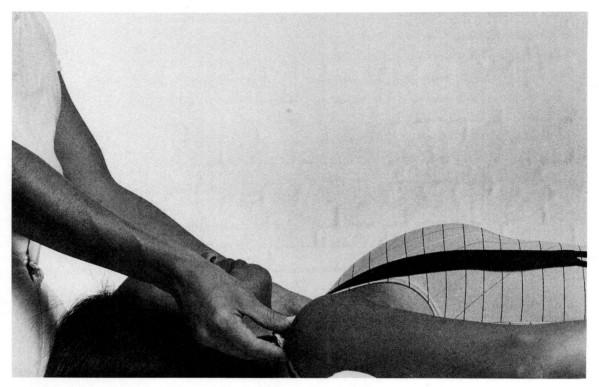

Vibration applied to the neck muscles. Headaches and tired shoulders are aided by the release of tight neck muscles. *Photo by Ebet Roberts.*

Kelp is a seaweed that grows up to 400 feet long. It is rich in vitamins and minerals and will give you a beauty boost inside and out. It makes a healthy bath, and provides extra iron when taken in capsule form. Kelp is used in toothpaste, food supplements, beauty masks, and as a natural food thickener.

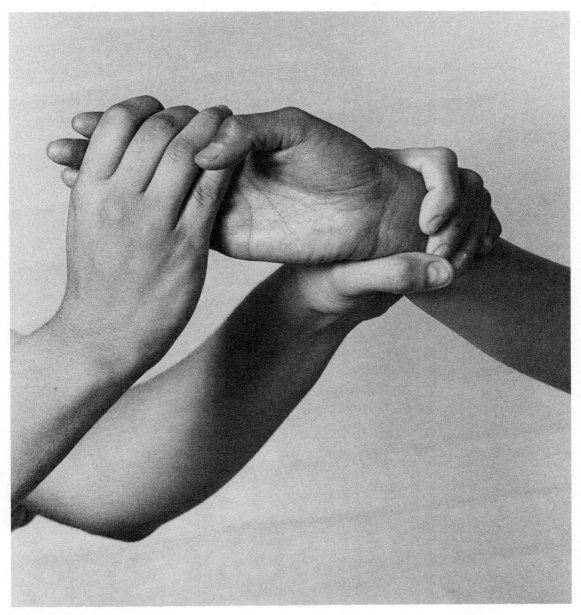

Range of motion applied to hands and wrists. Using both hands—one holding the wrist, the other grasping the fingers—rotate the axis of the wrist joint five times in each direction. This is an especially useful technique for players of golf and all racquet sports.

Visualization

Using your mind to assist your body in activities is more than possible! Visualization is creating images in your mind that are related to your desired result. By creating the desired circumstances in your mind, a mind-body connection is established. This connection will enhance any activity you pursue. For example, patients with lower-back pain were given a special visualization exercise to create the image of floating clouds in their minds. Their entire bodies began to relax, and thus the lower-back muscles followed. Golf pro Arnold Palmer says that before every shot he creates a successful shot in his mind.

The best thing about all these processes is that they can be used together. It seems that they share a common language and purpose. Their goal is one: to treat you to a healing, healthful and enjoyable experience. And since the body responds to water in total harmony, understanding something about the way water works, how the body works and about the other techniques that help facilitate its actions will increase its benefits.

Now comes the best part: the different ways of using water for feeling your best. In the chapters that follow, we will discuss water therapies—whirlpools, saunas, pressurized showers, water massage, packs, therapeutic baths and other techniques—that will provide you with hours of pleasure. Use them, enjoy them and share them with your family and friends.

Water Classifications		
very cold	32°– 56°F	(0°–13.3°C)
cold	56°– 65°F	(13.3°–18.3°C)
cool	65°– 75°F	(18.3°–23.9°C)
neutral	75°– 92°F	(23.9°–33.3°C)
warm	98°–104°F	(36.1°–40°C)
hot	104°–	(40°–)

Benefits of Hydrotherapy

Water has a quality called the "k" factor that makes it highly therapeutic for the human body:

increases circulation

tones skin

unclogs pores

reduces toxicity in the blood

calms nerves

helps uplift emotions

releases negative emotions

harmonizes and organizes body functions

reduces aches and pains

reduces swelling

provides body with nutrients

regulates body temperature

cleanses pores, skin and hair

heats a chilled body

offers relief to tight or arthritic joints

lubricates muscles and tissues

satisfies feelings of thirst

aids in a variety of beauty treatments, including those to soften skin and eliminate varicosity, cellulite, premature facial lines

provides an overall sense of well-being.

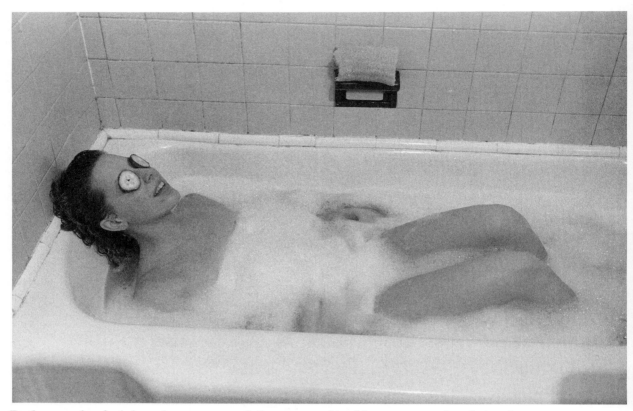

Baths—and a facial pack—are one of the most enjoyable ways to relax from the tensions of a busy day. See Chapter 9 for how to make a pack for complete relaxation and a better complexion.

3

THERAPEUTIC BATHS

Baths, in contrast with doctors' visits and medicine, are a cost-saving and easy way to soothe and relax a tired body. They also deodorize and open pores for healthier skin. Bathing is divided into several categories:

- bathing for cleanliness
- medical bathing
- bathing for relaxation
- religious and ceremonial bathing
- beauty bathing

Many cultures have used bathing for ritual and ceremonial purposes, as well as for health and beauty. History shows us that special bath chambers and large bathtubs were used. Often, large bathhouses were used for social gatherings and the discussion of worldly matters. Their tranquil environment provided the perfect atmosphere for these activities.

Throughout the world, there are some people who even today use baths as a religious or ceremonial experience. Their cleansing and purifying qualities no doubt play a significant role in these experiences. Many religions call for bathing before, after or during the observance of ceremonies. The ancient Hebrews, for example, believed it was important to bathe themselves before most religious ceremonies. The ancient Egyptians made the bath into a festive occasion, used to beautify, cleanse and for ritual purposes. Hindus consider the Ganges River sacred and come to bathe in its waters to purify themselves. The sick come to bathe in its waters, hoping it will cure their aches and pains. Christians celebrate a newborn's arrival or a person's entrance into the faith with a bath called baptism, in which the person is immersed in water.

Archaeologists have found the remains of baths in the ruins of many ancient civilizations. The ruins of the first public baths are believed to be about 4500 years old, and were located just outside of Pakistan. In ancient Rome, only the very wealthy could afford private bathrooms, but the Romans did build public bathhouses in nearly every city of the Empire. Many had marble floors and columns, hand-painted ceilings and many statues. The baths of Caracalla in Rome, built in the third century, could hold up to 1600 bathers at a time. During the Middle Ages in Europe, bathing declined in popularity. Public bathhouses were called ''stews,'' and bathing was called ''stewing'' because bathers often sat in hot water.

After recognizing its many benefits, most cultures have made bathing a part of their medical philosophy. Elegant bathhouses offering hot water, cold showers and plunging pools are not uncommon. For hundreds of years, people have visited health resorts called ''spas'' for medical baths. Most spas are located on the site of natural springs that yield bubbling heated or mineral water that is believed to have medicinal qualities.

Bathers sit in a tub that contains water. Soap combines with the water to remove bacteria, dead skin, dirt and body oils. The soap forms a thin layer around particles of dirt and suspends the particles in water until they are rinsed away. Bathing is beneficial in keeping the body healthy. Taking a bath in hot water that ranges from about 98°F to 112°F relaxes muscles, enlarges blood vessels near the surface of the skin and improves circulation. Warm baths that range from about 90°F to 97°F (32°–36°C) may help to relieve sleepiness and ease tension. Cold baths of less than 75°F (24°C) can reduce swelling. Whirlpool baths and water massages have been used successfully to treat arthritis, rheumatism and bone and muscle injuries.

Bathing for relaxation or pleasure is popular in many countries. In Japan, for example, people wash *before* soaking in a tub of hot water because the tub is used only for relaxation. During the 1970s in the U.S., hot tubs became popular and fashionable. Today, their use is in constant growth. A hot tub is a large tub in which two or more people soak in steaming, hot water. Some hot tubs are outdoors. They are equipped with a heater, filter and pump. The pump is used to circulate the water. Often, fragrant oils or special herbs are added for sensory stimulation.

One way to create sensory stimulation yourself is to boil one pint of water and add two tablespoons of peppermint tea and two tablespoons of camomile tea. Turn down the flame and let the brew simmer for about fifteen minutes. Strain the liquid through a cheesecloth (or a wooden or metal strainer). Add the liquid to your bathwater as the water is running.

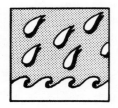

THE BATHROOM

Statistics show an ever-increasing interest in the bathroom among new homeowners. Home buyers are paying more attention to it when considering their needs. Some think of their home bathroom as special and almost sacred. Bathrooms can provide a tranquil sanctuary for family members, and you can do more with this space than you probably realize.

> Americans spent over 2.5 billion dollars on bathrooms and related facilities in 1986.

Colors, fragrances and practical needs are all to be considered when designing your bathroom's interior. Here is a list that you may find helpful in putting together your own bathroom environment:

reading rack or shelf
aromatic oils or fragrant incense
air purifier or ionizer
mirrors

plants and flowers

hot tub or whirlpool

massage-type shower head

soothing but vital colors on walls

supply of natural bath products

floor heater

natural lighting whenever possible

loofah and natural brushes

ample shelf or cabinet space

nonslip surface or rubber mat for tub

properly working floor scale

artwork, crafts or ocean designs to enhance atmosphere

The colors in your bathroom may be more important than you think. Colors can affect your body and your moods. While light colors reflect light and make surfaces appear larger and farther apart, dark colors absorb light and make the room seem smaller. Keep these remarks in mind as you plan your bath environment:

Red—stimulates, excites, increases energy and warms (not to be used when headaches, anger or inflammation are present)

Yellow—stimulates, warms, helps promote good digestion, clears overworked mind to allow for renewed mental capacity

Green—heals, nourishes, cools, vitalizes, creates harmony with nature, balances emotions

Blue—relaxes muscles, focuses thoughts, cools, instills a sense of tranquility and peace

Violet—soothes, calms, allows the mind to meditate

The choices in tubs today are wide. Tubs can be round, square, antique, on a platform, recessed, large or small—it's your choice. Natural fiber bath towels and washcloths come in a variety of sizes and are preferred over synthetic ones. They will, in the long run, treat your skin better, both stimulating it and letting it breathe.

As you can see, just stretching your imagination can produce hours of good health, beauty and pleasure without even leaving your bathroom.

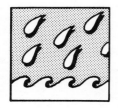

THE BATHING EXPERIENCE

Never should you be afraid to experiment with your baths. Try, for example, adding some rose petals, or a tablespoon of yogurt to the water. Yogurt both softens skin and adds a delicious flavor to a bath. For a relaxing bubble bath try mixing powdered milk to your water. If you use a commercial bubble-bath mix, make sure that it does not contain harmful chemicals or mineral oil, which will leave the skin dry and rob it of vitamins. Just let your mind run free when it comes to the rewards of a bath.

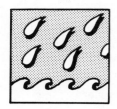

HERBAL BATHS

Herbal baths or medicated baths provide the luxury of feeling good as they offer medicinal benefits. These baths can be hot, cold or neutral. The herbal solution may consist of herbs or flowers. Herbal baths also utilize tea infusions, essential oils and various sea products that penetrate the skin to engage in the healing experience. They can have a profound regenerating effect on your body.

Actions of the herbal bath are:

relief from tight, sore muscles

increases vitality

enhances circulation

reduces fever

helps mend bones

lubricates stiff joints

softens and beautifies skin tissues

acts as an anesthetic

acts as an antiseptic

cleanses skin, removes dead skin cells

helps recovery from illness

strengthens body

Any substance that has healing properties can be added to your bathwater. Below are a list of herbs, flowers or oils that may be added to your bath:

SAGE—clears the memory, stimulates hair growth, stimulates energy

COMFREY—helps mend bones, relieves rheumatism, soothes minor aches and pains, provides nutrients for improved circulation

SEA SALT—cleanses, soothes skin, relieves minor aches

APPLE CIDER VINEGAR—rejuvenates and helps build up body's resistance, removes toxins from skin

SPIRULINA—simulates ocean (its blue-green color is reminiscent of a dip in the tropical waters), adds vitamins and minerals to bathwater.

KELP—soothes skin, relaxes entire body, provides nutrients for good skin tone

WINTERGREEN—the aromatic way to reproduce the great fresh outdoors. Invigorates, gives the body strength and vitality

CAMOMILE—relaxes, soothes, beautifies. Because of its fragrant aroma, appealing flowers and therapeutic value, I recommend that you keep a batch of fresh camomile flowers in your bathroom—it is a subtle but rewarding herbal

ROSE AND JASMINE—the two most used flowers in beauty mixtures; both have high vibrational qualities and should be considered when relaxation, soothing, calming and softening are desired. Rose oil or jasmine oil can be added to any bath for their fragrant qualities

There are a number of ways to prepare herbal baths:

1. Make a tea infusion by boiling some water. To each cup of water, add one tablespoon of bathing herbs. Cover and allow the mixture to simmer for approximately fifteen minutes. Different herbs will need a

little longer to simmer. Strain the liquid through a fine strainer and pour the liquid into your bath. The water in your bath can be cold or hot, although hot water works best with the qualities of herbs.

2. Place herbs in an old cotton sock and place the sock under or over the faucet in the tub. Turn on the water and allow the hot water to run through the sock and over the herbs. Essential oils may be added directly to the water in minute amounts. When using sea salt, spirulina or the like, you may add it directly to the bathwater.

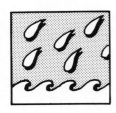 ## FULL HOT BATHS

This type of bath is useful to sedate and relax the body. It also helps to relieve minor aches and pains and eliminate toxins from the skin's surface. The bathwater should be as hot as the body can tolerate for optimal effectiveness. During the bath, it is important to run fresh hot water as the water cools.

Actions of a full hot bath:

alleviates pain

reduces muscle spasm

relieves congestion

relieves constipation

stretches tight muscles

relieves bronchitis

relieves sciatica

relieves hemorrhoids

rejuvenates body

relieves bursitis

helps reduce anger and worry

relaxes and calms body

relieves arthritis

stimulates and soothes inflamed gall bladder

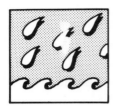

RELAXING BATHS

For a relaxing bath, make the water warm and comfortable. It will help soothe and calm your body. It is especially helpful after a stress-filled or energy-packed day. The relaxing bath sedates the muscles and helps clear the mind for a peaceful inner feeling (remember, however, that the relaxing bath is effective as a temporary solution and is *not* the answer to long-term stress control). This bath is also a great way to facilitate mental concentration. It offers a good space in which to ''cool out'' and simply ''ponder life.''

1. Fill the tub. Always run hot water first and then add cold water until the desired temperature is achieved.

2. Use a pillow or rolled towel on which to rest your head and neck. Sit in the tub upright for a few moments, finally resting your head against the back, with your body extended as fully as possible. Once your body is resting, try the following relaxation exercise: Inhale slowly, taking in as much air as possible; hold your breath for a count of five, and then exhale twice, as slowly as you inhaled. Repeat this several times. Slowly close your eyes and allow your entire body to sink down into the tub in a state of total relaxation.

As the water begins to cool, run more hot water in. If you want an herbal bath, add herbs to your relaxing bath. A tea infusion of lavender or rose flowers is wonderful.

During the relaxing bath, a blue or violet light bulb may help set the mood by creating a relaxing and calming atmosphere. And, finally, soothing music can be used. For a very deep relaxing bath, add two tablespoons of hops to the bathwater.

To relieve muscular tension and minor aches and pains, draw a very hot bath. Add two tablespoons of sea salt to the water and one drop of wintergreen oil or peppermint oil. During the bath, massage the muscles or perform some of the bathtub exercises (see pages 58–75) and follow the relaxation instructions for the relaxing bath. Try using a visualization exercise in which you feel your tight muscles relaxing and releasing their tension.

It is important to obtain a state of near-total relaxation during any kind of bath. The relaxation will allow you to involve your mind in the process, thus enhancing any positive benefits. You can actually help a muscle to relax by using the power of your mind. After all, it is the brain that ultimately gives the muscle the command to move. Use your breathing to help soothe your tense muscles.

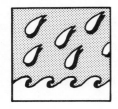 ## *FULL COLD BATHS*

Unlike full hot baths, which relax the body, full cold baths act as a tonic and rejuvenator by constricting rather than expanding blood vessels. Cold water awakens, enlivens and vitalizes.

Actions of the full cold bath are:

stimulates body

acts as a tonic to the entire system

strengthens the immune system

creates a state of vitality

helps relieve rheumatism

lowers fevers

provides a feeling of exhilaration

rejuvenates

stimulates clogged pores

Before taking a cold bath, take a hot shower, then immerse yourself into the full tub of cold water. Massage the body vigorously. Once again, the water should be as cold as your body can tolerate. Remain in it for at least three minutes. The cold bath is also great after a sauna or hot bath.

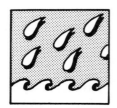

TONIC FRICTION BATHS

Tonic friction baths have benefits similar to those of massage. This bath can be used on the entire body, or just on a local area. During the bath, vigorous rubbing and kneading are used for toning and stimulating the circulation. The benefits are especially useful to a person who is in a weak state of health, or recovering from an illness. The tonic friction bath's main claim to fame is that it stimulates the entire circulatory system. As it restores body tone, it also helps build immune system response and reduces fever.

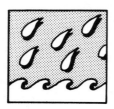

BRUSH MASSAGE BATHS

These baths make use of a brush or loofah to brush and firmly rub the body during the bath. Brushing the body is routine after a sauna as an aid to proper circulation.

The loofah is a natural sea sponge that can be purchased at most drugstores and health-food stores. It has therapeutic benefits for the skin, as it acts as an exfoliate, washing away dead skin cells and stimulating the surface layer of the skin. When selecting a brush, make sure it contains natural hair or silk bristles. These will not damage your skin.

Actions of the brush massage bath are:

relieves asthma
removes dead cells
unclogs pores
relieves varicose veins

helps break up cellulite
body tonic and vitalizer
enhances circulation

The following is a suggested way to enjoy the benefits of the brush massage bath. First, soap the entire body with a natural soap. Peppermint soap or olive-oil soap are good choices. Dip the brush or loofah into the warm or hot water and scrub the skin for two to five minutes. As you stroke the skin, use circular motions until the skin is red and the body feels invigorated. End the bath with a warm shower, gradually reducing the water temperature until it becomes cool.

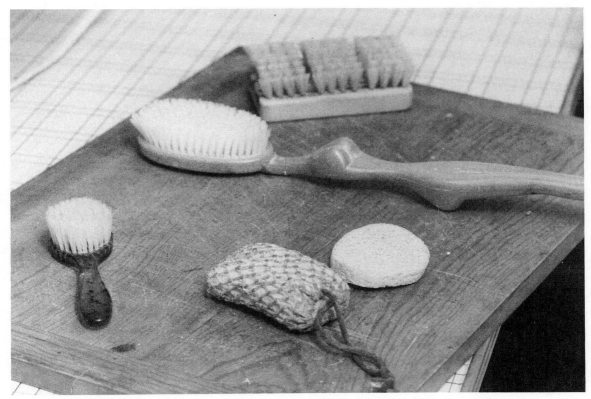

Natural bristle brushes offer the best way of cleaning and beautifying your skin. A variety of products made from natural substances including seaweed and natural fiber may also be used.

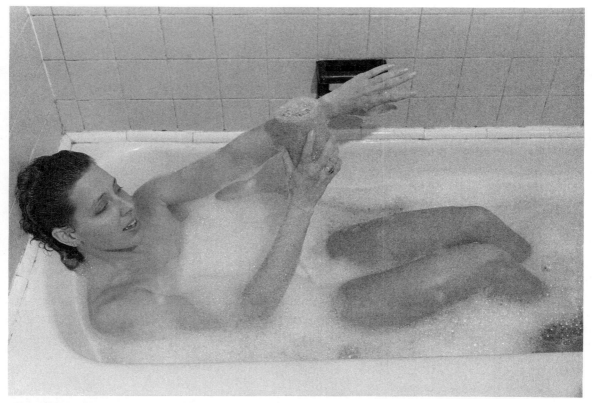

Scrubbing with seaweed soap and natural cloth enhances surface circulation, which will give you a more beautiful complexion.

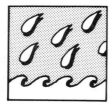 ## SITZ BATHS

This type of bath uses only five to ten inches of water. The buttocks are just about covered. A hip or half-bath extends to the hips and partially up to the lower abdomen. They are effective because the water acts only on a localized section of the body.

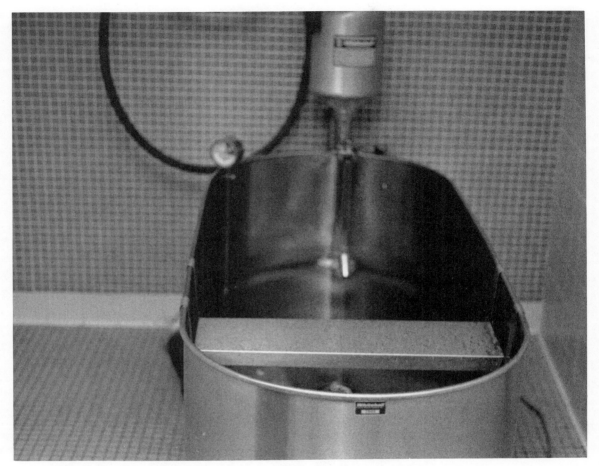

An example of a sitz bath. Hot water acts on all pelvic and abdominal areas. It is best to begin the bath with water temperature at body temperature, 92°F–98°F. Gradually develop your tolerance to 120°F.

A sitting or kneeling cold bath daily will build resistance and vitality. Immerse only the buttocks, upper thighs and lower abdomen in the water. This is achieved by using either a hospital sitz bath or a bidet attachment, or by sitting in an ordinary bathtub in six to ten inches of cold water, with your legs elevated or propped up on a pillow. If you use a hot sitz bath, try putting a cold compress on your head. This will enhance the benefits greatly.

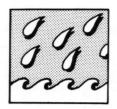

ALTERNATING HOT AND COLD BATHS

These baths have a special magic all their own. The mixing together of these two elements activates all functions of the body. Usually starting with hot water and ending with cold water, alternating baths massage the circulatory system, first expanding then constricting it. This inner pulsating experience helps break up harmful toxins in the blood to enhance your overall health.

Actions of the alternating hot and cold bath are:

relieves abdominal congestion

relieves prostate inflammation

relieves hemorrhoids

strengthens male sexual ability

sedates and rejuvenates entire system

increases circulation

acts as a tonic

enlivens, vitalizes

It is usually best to sit first in a tub of hot water for up to five minutes, then in a tub of cold water for one minute (by running hot water first, then cold). Try to alternate this process at least five or six times. Always end the rotation with cool water.

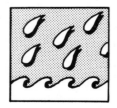

LOCALIZED BATHS

An *eye bath* rinses the eyes and cleanses them. This bath will also help to relieve sensitive nerve endings and tissue in the eye area, removing pressure from it.

Actions of the eye bath are:

reduces irritation
reduces inflammation
reduces tissue swelling
removes foreign objects from the eye
allows you to see things more clearly
soothes tired eyes

Simply purchase an eye cup from a pharmacy or drugstore. Fill it with water that is at body temperature. You will know instantly if it is

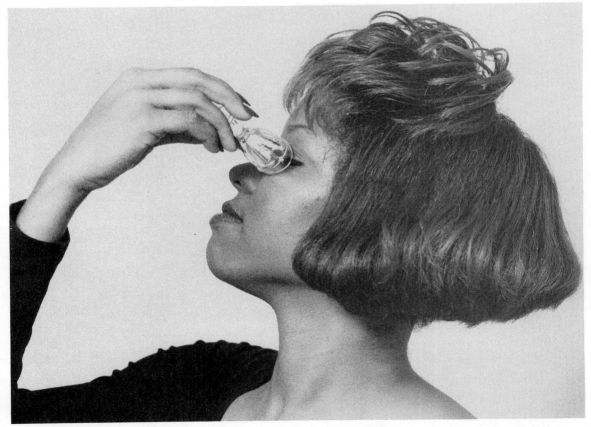

An old-fashioned eye cup with plain water can be used to rinse and soothe tired eyes. Be sure that the solution is free of loose particles before using.

too hot or too cold. (Make sure the water is pure spring water or distilled.) Rinse the eye several times. If you use an herb, such as eyebright, in your solution, be sure to strain all fine particles out of the solution before using it. Often, eye irritations cause us to have a foggy vision of our lives.

Ear baths (which you should *always* consult your doctor before attempting) function very much like eye baths. You may purchase a commercial ear syringe from a pharmacy or drugstore.

Wash out the ear with a warm water solution (spring, distilled or tap water may be used), or use an herbal such as mullein. The ear syringe will pump the solution into the ear and suction it out.

Actions of the ear bath are:

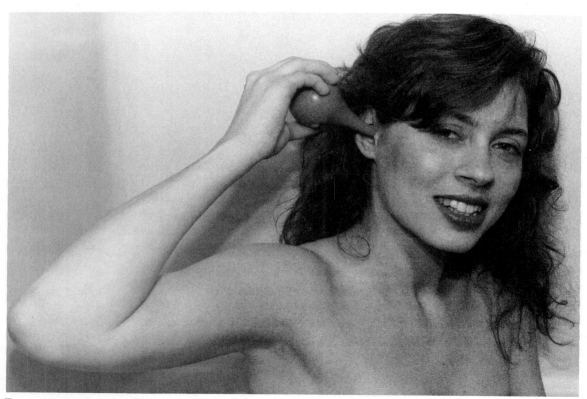

Be very gentle when using an ear squeeze.

removes foreign matter from the ear

unclogs air pockets

soothes irritation

breaks up minor wax deposits

The *head bath* involves only the head. By immersing this area in water, circulation is concentrated here to help achieve the desired results. Herbal infusions of peppermint or sage can be added to the bathwater to enhance its benefits to the head and hair. Immerse the head in warm or cold water, as the situation calls for.

Actions of the head bath are:

relieves most types of headache (cool water)

breaks up head congestion in colds, etc. (warm to hot water)

relieves worry and anger (cold water)

counters the effects of excessive thinking (alternating hot and cold water)

restores circulation to head area (alternating hot and cold water)

improves memory (alternating hot and cold water)

stimulates hair growth (alternating hot and cold water)

improves stimulation in the face (cold to cool water)

Head baths are not commonly used; however, I find them a valuable part of a total hydrotherapy program. They can be especially useful to students and business people who need to think and make decisions constantly.

Foot baths localize the circulation and place additional healing energy in that area. This type of bath is one of the best for your body. A good foot bath can send healing energy throughout your entire body. When the foot is stimulated, reflex points that correspond to other parts of the body are also stimulated.

Walking in a foot or so of cold water will stimulate and rejuvenate the entire body, while walking back and forth in a foot of hot water will help to relax it. Of course, if your body is overheated, angry or upset, cold water is best; if you are experiencing chills or a cold, warm water is best.

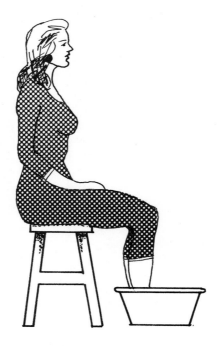

At the end of the day, soak your pains away. Fill a large tub full of warm water and herbs, and immerse your feet in it for about fifteen minutes.

Actions of the foot bath include:

increases circulation

warms cold feet and toes

beautifies feet

helps dissolve and soften corns and calluses

soothes tired feet

calms nerves

relieves varicose veins

overcomes general weakness

increases vitality

aids in ankle swelling

reduces high blood pressure

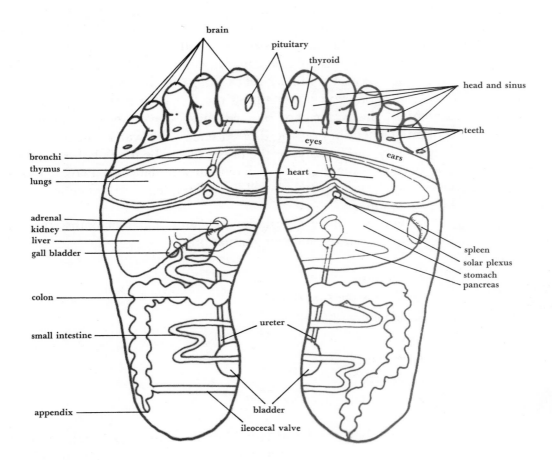

After a good foot soak, try a foot massage. By using finger pressure on the points in the drawing above, you can stimulate various areas of the body. This technique is known as reflexology.

For an effective foot bath, walk and soak in warm water flavored with the herb or oil of your choice for five to ten minutes. Some companies produce a commercial foot massager and bath that may be used while sitting, reading or watching TV. Walking along the seashore, in water reaching your ankles, is a natural form of the foot bath and adds the therapeutic benefits of organic water. Another pleasurable experience, with wide-reaching benefits, is walking on hot sand. The sand will both massage and stimulate reflex points in the feet.

Still another way of bathing the feet is in a running bath. In this foot bath, the water (hot or cold) moves over the foot in a constant motion. Depending on the desired effect, the water can move over the foot rapidly and heavily, or the pressure can be much lighter and slower. Heavy, quick-moving water will tend to stimulate and increase the body's action; slow, light pressure will have a tendency to sedate and relax the body's action.

If you are using alternating hot and cold foot baths, their action may help you in the following situations:

insomnia

swollen ankles (sprain)

headache

low vitality

toothache

congestion

constipation

For the best results when taking alternating foot baths, soak in hot water (100°F–110°F) for three minutes, then in cold water (60°F) for thirty seconds. Repeat the rotation three times, ending with cool water.

The *hand soak or bath* has many of the same benefits as the foot bath. It is said that hands are an extension of the heart. Tension, anger, jealousy and fear will lead to arthritic pain in the hands and wrists. Often, the way we touch others may be an initial clue about our internal feelings. A warm heart will lead to a warm touch.

Hands are filled with sensory feelers. They hold on to things and they are also responsible for letting go of unwanted energies in our life. Finally, hands are used for expressing love.

Actions of the hand bath are:

relieves writer's, typist's or other occupational cramps
relieves arthritis in wrist or fingers
warms cold fingertips
improves overall circulation
beautifies and softens hands
strengthens nails

For the above results, soak the hands in hot water to which you may add rosemary or sage tea. Soak hands for thirty seconds to three

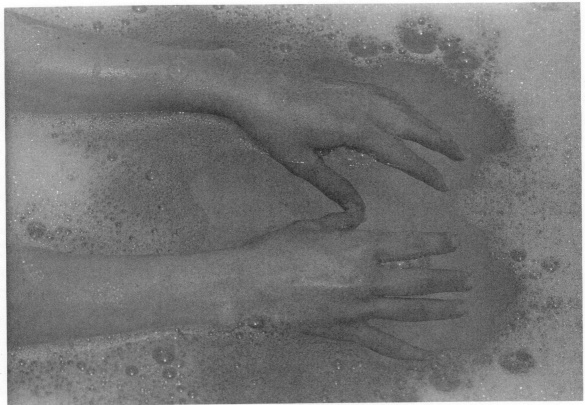

A good hand soak can ease away the day's cares.

minutes. Repeat this at least twice a day. Massage the hands and rotate the wrists at the end of the soak.

To improve circulation in the hands or wrists, try adding one-half teaspoon of cayenne pepper to two glasses of water for a dynamite energizer. When the circulation is improved, nutrients and healing energies are generated that help almost any condition in the hand, fingers or wrist.

Try this delightful hot oil soak for more attractive hands and feet. Heat one cup of olive oil in a pot. When the oil is cool enough to allow you to immerse your hand or foot (but still warm enough to be therapeutic), soak for three minutes. Repeat with the other hand or foot. (If you have to reheat the oil between dips, by all means do so. Make the oil as warm as you can tolerate it. Be careful not to spill hot oil on yourself; use caution in handling the pot.)

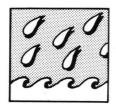

BEAUTY BATHS

Beauty baths are both therapeutic and pleasurable. Since our skin gets water-saturated, when we bathe vital beautifying elements have a free ride into the cells where physical beauty originates.

There are many prepackaged beauty products on the market today. When you select them, make sure you stay as close as possible to purity and quality. Be sure to read the labels for synthetic ingredients, additives and harmful chemicals. Just because the label says ''all natural'' doesn't mean it is. Avoid anything that will irritate or inflame the skin and products that are malodorous or that are to be blended with ingredients that have spoiled. Some synthetic products will actually rob the skin of valuable nutrients and dry it out.

Flowers, exotic oils and herbs can help you have the ultimate beauty bath. First, select your favorite fragrance. Add one or two drops to a warm bath. Add two drops of pure olive oil to the water. (There are also a number of fine commercial bath oils on the market.) And, finally, pour one cup of camomile tea infusion into the bathwater. This bath will soften your skin while rejuvenating and moisturizing it. If you want to use colors in your bath, try floating pink flower petals in the water, or use pink bath crystals.

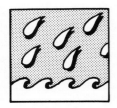

ROMANTIC BATHS

Of course, the idea of what a romantic moment is and what constitutes intimacy varies from person to person and from couple to couple. The selection of music, choice of fragrance and decor in the environment all play a role in setting the stage for a passionate, caring experience in which two hearts interact for the evening. The romantic bath is an intimate way of experiencing a memorable and pleasurable exchange with your romantic partner.

To create a special floral decor, sprinkle one teaspoon each of rose and lavender in your warm bathwater. Use a cotton cloth; or you may want to invest in a dollar's worth of silk fabric that you have folded into squares. With a small amount of soap, wash your mate from head to toe. For a light sensual touch, use a liquid soap such as castile (available in pure flavors). Remember, go slowly, caressing the body as you lather and stroke it gently. Keep the cloth soaking wet as you do this. On the back and chest, try using small circular motions that get larger as you continue. Once again, take your time, massaging with a caring sensitivity that will be realized by your partner.

Feet and hands are important during the romantic bath. Everybody loves a good foot massage! Do not forget the fingertips and the toes. Massage the entire foot and the entire hand. You might also try massaging the head and hair with your hands. To rinse each part, simply fill the cloth with water and manually rinse it off. Let your partner relax and enjoy the experience as much as possible. Next time, it's your turn.

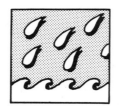

ENERGIZING BATHS

The cold foot bath is a basic energizer. Since it combines the properties of foot massage, cold water and herbals, it can be rejuvenating to the entire system. Use a commercial foot bath, a foot tub, or even your regular bathtub.

Sitting in a chair, place both feet in the cold water. Place one-half teaspoon of cayenne pepper into the water. Cayenne is one of the world's best stimulants, pushing the blood through the body as it enhances circulation. In place of cayenne (but not nearly as effective), you can use a tea infusion of peppermint, sage or wintergreen.

Soak your feet in the foot bath for at least fifteen minutes. During each fifteen-minute period, take your feet out of the water at least three times for a minute or so each time. As the water warms up, add ice or ice-cold water to maintain the temperature.

Finally, when your feet are out of the water, massage the areas shown in the chart using small, circular motions.

At the end of the cold foot bath, rinse the feet in warm water, then in cool water. Dry them vigorously with a heavy cotton towel. To soften them, rub a thin coat of pure (cold-pressed) olive oil on the feet and ankles.

If you have heart disease, varicose veins or high blood pressure, check with your physician before taking a cold foot bath.

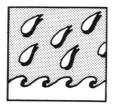

BATHTUB EXERCISES

The therapeutic powers of water are wonderful. Water offers general relief for back and neck pain, one of the most common ailments known

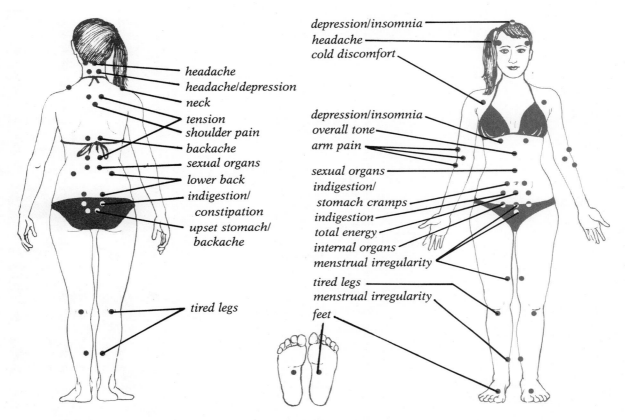

Important pressure points.

in the Western Hemisphere. Also, the nagging irritation of arthritic joint pain may be relieved in the bathtub. Both prevention and timely treatment will allay muscular problems and premature arthritic conditions.

Actions of bathtub exercises are:

increase circulation
help joints gain wider range of movement and flexibility
break up toxins for release through the skin
strengthen and tone body for optimal health and beauty
provide overall sense of poise and well-being

Chart 1 Occupational Problems:
White Collar Workers

BODY PROBLEM	WATERWORKS	Architects	Desk workers/clerks	Executives/Managers	Lawyers	Receptionists	Secretaries/Admin. Assts.	Students	Writers/Editors/Journalists
Atrophy in stomach muscles/fast food syndrome	Relaxing Bath and Juices	■		■					
Back problems	Bathtub Exercises and Packs on Lower Back	■		■	■		■		■
Cramps in hand/arthritis	Cold/Hot Compresses on Wrist		■		■	■			
Eyestrain	Eye Bath			■				■	■
General muscular atrophy	Swimming	■	■					■	
Headaches	Cold Head Compresses		■	■	■		■		
Heart disorders	Relaxing Bath and Juices			■			■		■
Lower back pain	Leg Lifts in Tub and Packs on Lower Back				■				■
Mental fatigue	Sauna and Bathtub Exercises		■	■				■	
Pain in wrist & upper arm	Cold/Hot Compresses on Wrist			■		■		■	
Shoulder pain	Bathtub Exercises	■	■	■			■		
Stiff neck	Neck and Throat Compresses		■				■		■
Stress overload	Steam				■		■	■	
Throat irritations	Localized Shower on Throat and Drink Fresh Water			■		■			■

Chart 2 Occupational Problems:
Trade Workers

BODY PROBLEM	WATERWORKS	Artists (studio)	Carpenters	Chefs/cooks	Construction workers	Drivers (cab, bus)/Pilots	Dry cleaners	Electricians	Firefighters	Jewelers	Painters	Photographers	Repairmen	Tailors
Backaches	Leg Lifts in Tub and Packs on Lower Back		■			■		■			■		■	■
Bruises/injuries	Herbal Bath			■										
Burns	Ice Therapy				■			■						
Eyestrain	Eye Bath and Eye Massage	■			■			■		■		■	■	
Finger pain and stiffness	Wrist Rotations	■								■			■	
Knee problems	Hot Knee Compresses	■												
Neck and shoulder problems	Shoulder Shrugs and Localized Shower					■		■			■	■	■	■
Nervous disorders	Whirlpool and Relaxing Bath					■			■					
Respiratory problems	Swimming and Sauna	■							■			■		
Skin disorders	Ice therapy and Herbal Sauna						■							
Stomach disorders	Herbal Teas and Fresh Fruits and Vegetables				■	■								
Tightness in jaw	Localized Shower and Ice Therapy											■		
Wrist problem	Wrist Rotations													■

Chart 3 Occupational Problems: Service Workers

BODY PROBLEM	WATERWORKS	Bank Tellers	Flight attendants	Haircutters	Librarians	Massage therapists	Physicians and nurses	Police officers	Postal workers	Sales personnel	Teachers	Telephone operators	Waiters
Back strain	Shoulder Shrugs and Relaxing Herbal Baths				X	X							X
Cramps in hand & fingers	Finger Exercises, Hand Soak, and Compresses on Wrist	X		X	X				X			X	
Eyestrain	Eye Bath	X			X				X			X	X
Foot & leg pains	Foot Bath, Knee Lifts in Tub, and Knee Compresses			X				X	X	X			X
Headaches	Ear Bath and Localized Shower to Neck and Back								X	X			
Neck	Shoulder Shrugs		X		X							X	
Overweight	Swimming							X	X				
Shoulder pain	Shoulder Shrug and Compresses to Shoulder	X	X	X		X			X			X	
Sore muscles	Sauna, Steam, and Whirlpool						X						
Stomach problems	Drink Fresh Juice and Fresh Water and Relaxing Bath								X	X	X		
Tension/nervousness	Whirlpool and Footbath						X	X	X				
Voice & throat problems	Neck and Throat Compresses, Drink Fresh Water									X	X		X

Chart 4 Occupational Problems: Performers

BODY PROBLEM	WATERWORKS	Actors	Athletes	Dancers	Musicians: wind instrument players	Musicians: string & percussion	Politicians	Vocalists	Radio & TV announcers
All types of musculoskeletal injuries	Localized Shower	■		■					
Backache	Whirlpool, Packs on Lower Back, Localized Shower		■				■		
Chest pain	Chest Compress	■	■		■				
Cramps in fingers	Wrist and Finger Exercises		■			■			
Cramps in legs	Ice Compresses to Legs and Ankles, Whirlpool		■	■					
Feet problems	Foot Baths and Foot Massage			■					
Lung and breathing problems	Chest Compresses	■	■		■		■	■	■
Problems with joints	Hot/Cold Compresses and Bathtub Exercises		■	■		■			
Shoulder pain	Localized Shower, Whirlpool, Sauna		■			■			
Stomach problems	Relaxing Baths		■						
Tension	Relaxing Baths	■	■				■		■
Throat problems	Steam, Hot Compresses, Localized Shower	■						■	■
Tightness in jaw	Hot Compresses, Localized Shower			■	■				
Voice Problems	Hot Compresses to Throat and Chest	■				■		■	■
Wrist problems	Wrist and Finger Exercises, Hand soak		■			■			

It is a myth that exercise should be painful to have beneficial results. Water exercises are always done gently and easily. Here are a few simple rules to remember:

- Never overextend a body part; stretch it to its natural limitation, and then stop.
- Never stretch to the point of intense pain.
- Move slowly and deliberately.
- Use a rubber mat in the tub to give you support.
- Breathe with the movement to allow your energy flow to help you.

Water allows the body to be buoyant, thus relieving it from the stress and strain of supporting itself. It absorbs the gravity of the body's weight. While your body is suspended in the water, you are more relaxed and thus more receptive to the benefits of bath exercises.

It is best to begin each exercise gradually and work up to a more intense movement. Also, it is imperative that you focus on your breathing. Breathing is the real key to a successful exercise program. As you breathe in, muscles contract; as you exhale, muscles relax and expand. So, be sure to breathe naturally and fluidly, in and out. You will see better results once you coordinate your breathing.

For these exercises, your bathwater should be between 80°F and 90°F. A twenty-minute bath will be sufficient. Some of the exercises will need to be repeated several times. Each time you repeat the same exercise, it is called a ''repetition,'' or ''rep.'' If, for example, you repeat a push-up four times, you have completed four reps. A set is a group of repetitions. Since reps are grouped together, sets tell you how many of these groups you will be performing. There is usually a rest period in between each set to allow the muscle to rest.

Make sure your bathroom is warm and as comfortable as possible. For an extra incentive, put on some music to exercise by. When doing the stretching exercises, hold them for at least ten seconds, and longer whenever you can.

The Bathtub Exercise Program

1. Standing stretch (this should be done before you enter the bath)—

Place both hands over your head. Breathe in and reach up, as though you are reaching for the stars (brace yourself and be careful not to slip). Stretch as far as you can. Do not move your feet or your legs; stretch only your arms, hands and upper body. Stretch as you inhale, hold for ten seconds, then relax as you exhale. Repeat the standing stretch three times, each time stretching a bit farther.

2. Neck rotations—Still standing, rotate your neck by dropping your head to your chest. Then, relax by inhaling and exhaling three times. Begin by turning the neck and head to the right, in complete circles. When starting, turn the neck in small, slow circles, and gradually allow the circles to get larger and larger. Rotate the neck on its full axis, experiencing a wide range of motion. Go slowly, there's no rush!

3. Shoulder shrugs—Now, slowly sit in the tub. Lift your shoulders up toward your ears, in a straight line with them. Shrug your shoulders (as if you don't know the answer) and hold for ten seconds. Repeat this three times. Once again, go slowly.

4. Foot rotations—These are great for tired feet or ankle sprains. Relax even farther into the water. Close your eyes and allow your body to feel the lightness it assumes in the water. Feel the buoyancy and flow with it. Focus your mind on your feet: Imagine a straight line of string from your head to your feet, connecting the two. Begin by rotating your left foot to the left as far as possible. These foot rotations are similar to neck rotations. Next, rotate your left foot as far as possible to the right. Repeat each direction at least eighteen times before changing to the right foot. Finally, point both feet toward your chest. Hold for at least ten seconds. Repeat this three times.

5. Toe flex—Flex your toes and squeeze them together. Hold the flexion for about ten seconds, then release. Repeat this three times.

6. Leg lifts—Grip the sides of the tub if you find that you need added support with this exercise. Inhale and lift your legs just a few inches from the bottom of the tub. Hold this position for approximately five seconds, then slowly bring your legs back down. Repeat three times with each leg.

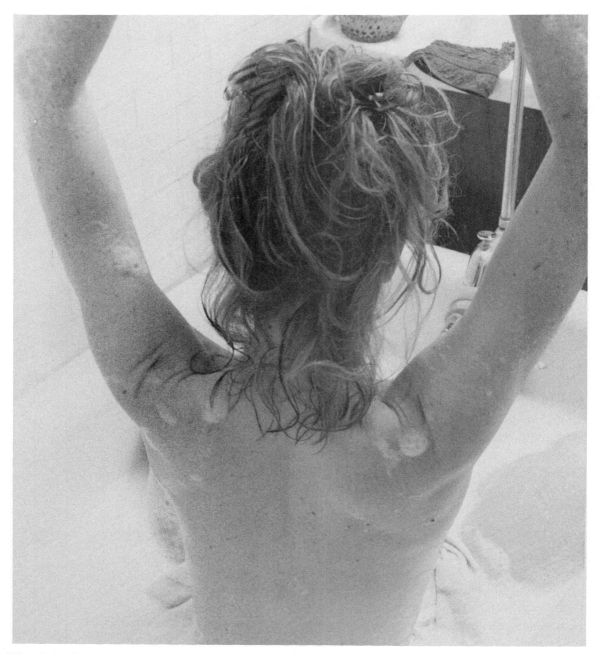

The Arm Stretch: Lift your arms straight up as if you were reaching for the ceiling. This exercise stretches your entire back and tones the neck and shoulders.

7. Knee lifts—Dip slightly into the tub, using the sides of the tub as a support. Bend your left knee toward your left shoulder as you slowly raise the foot, then the entire left leg, until it is straight up (or as horizontal as possible). Slowly lower it until it is on the tub floor. Inhale as you lift, exhale as you lower the leg. Repeat at least three times with each knee.

8. Knee bends—Sit up against the back of the tub. Bend your left knee toward your chest and hold it for a count of at least ten. (Your right leg should remain relaxed and straight.) When you release, slowly straighten out your leg, using the water as natural resistance. Repeat the same with the right leg.

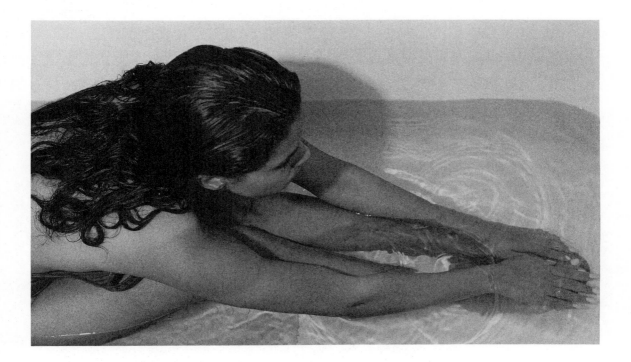

Bend and Stretch: Bend over at the waist, reaching as far as you can toward your toes. This stretches the entire body.

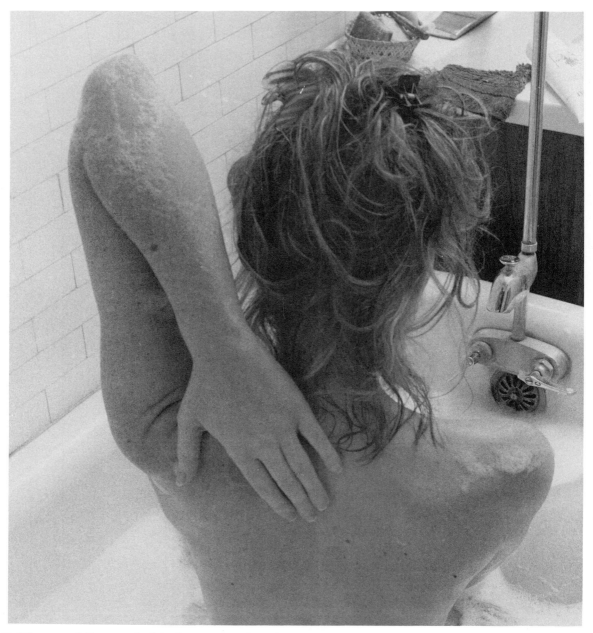

Fold your right arm behind your head and move your right shoulder toward your back. Hold the position for a few seconds, then release. Repeat with the left arm. This is a muscle stretch that relieves tension around the shoulder blade.

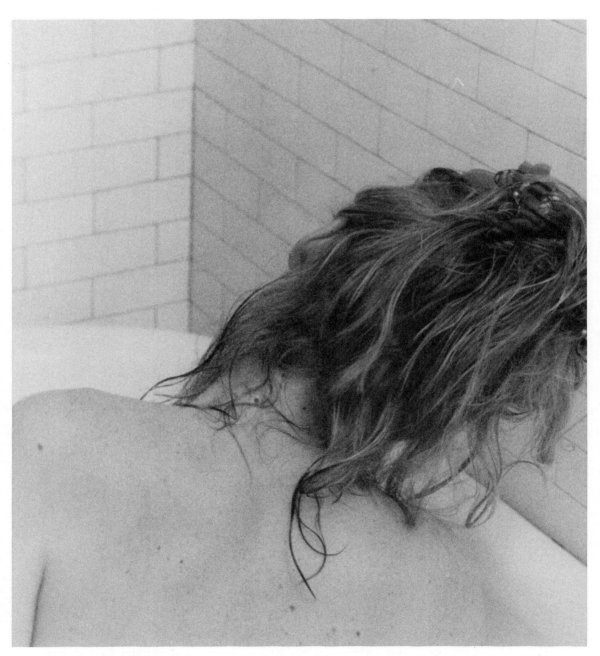

Neck Rotation Exercise: Tilt the neck to each side to relieve tension and stress in the neck, shoulders and upper back. It also helps to take pressure off the upper spine.

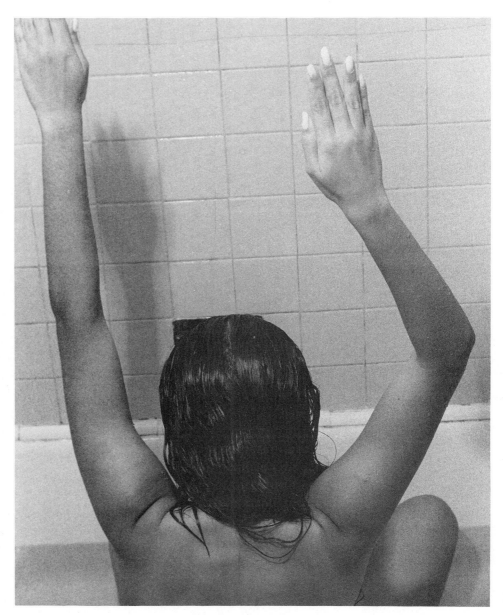

The Shoulder Shrug: Shrug shoulders up toward your ears, hold and inhale deeply for approximately five seconds, then exhale. Repeat five times, then relax totally. This is marvelous for relieving the day's tension in your neck, throat, chest and upper back.

9. Hand toner—Put both hands underwater and squeeze them closed. Quickly open and close them, as though you were trying to grasp a handful of water. Repeat this exercise at least eighteen times, in three sets of five each.

10. Back bend—Sitting up in the tub, bring your knees to your chest. Inhale, hold your breath and bend forward. When you have reached your maximum stretch, rest and exhale. As your muscles relax, you can again reach a new maximum by stretching farther. Repeat this three times.

As you can see, the ordinary bath is not so ordinary after all. Its benefits are far-reaching. They touch our physical, mental, social and recreational lives, offering many ways to help make each a more rewarding experience.

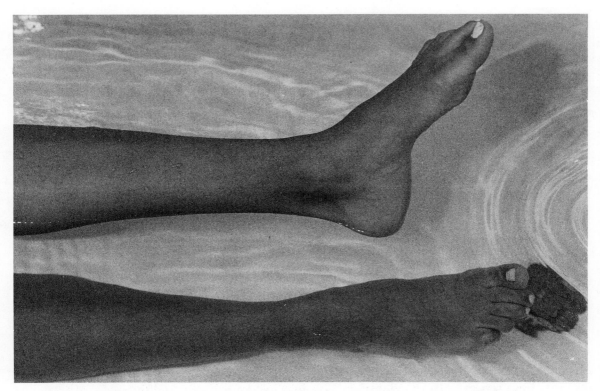

Foot Rotation: Rotate your right foot clockwise ten times, then counterclockwise ten times. Repeat with your left foot.

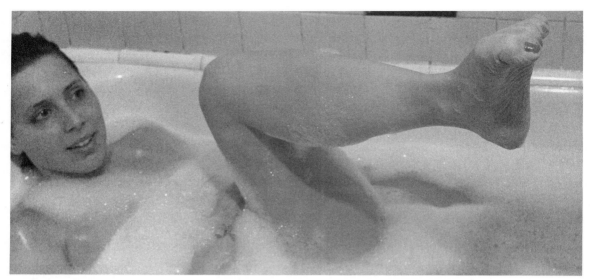

Toe Curls: Curl the toes of your right foot, hold for five seconds, then release. Repeat three times. Do the same with your left foot. This soothes tired feet and stimulates foot joints.

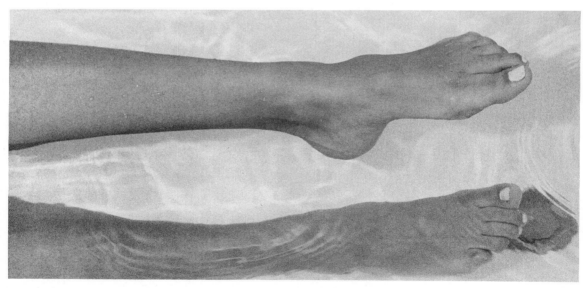

Leg Lift: Lift your left leg approximately one foot out of the water, hold for a few seconds, then repeat with the right leg. You will feel your thighs tighten immediately. This will tone your thighs and tighten your buttocks.

Try singing while you do the leg-lift exercise. If you don't have a great singing voice, this will at least give you shapely legs!

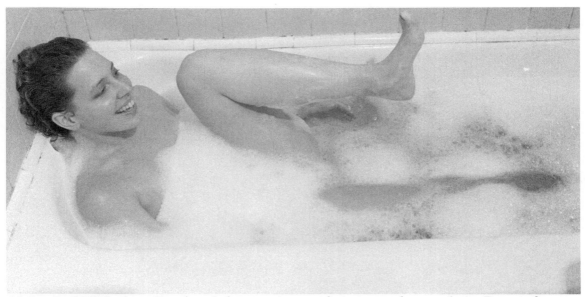

Abdominal Tightener: Bend each knee, one at a time, toward your chest. Repeat five times with each leg. This will tighten your stomach and abdominal muscles.

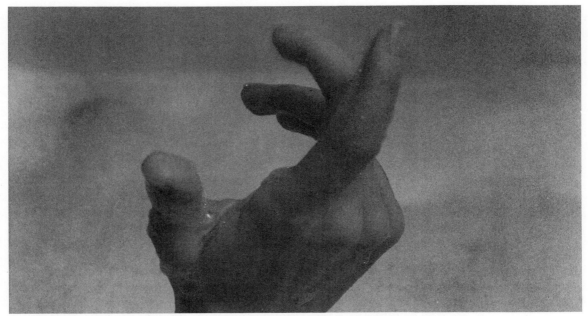

To exercise your fingers, rotate each one clockwise five times and then counterclockwise five times. This will stimulate the circulation to your fingertips.

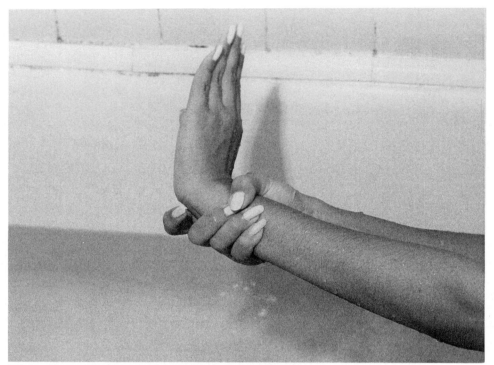

Wrist Rotation: Rotate your right wrist clockwise ten times, then counterclockwise ten times. Repeat with your left wrist. This will prevent painful joints, increase your range of motion and may help increase circulation to relieve arthritic pain.

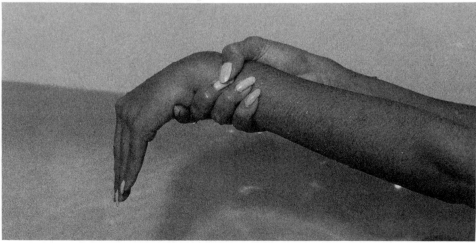

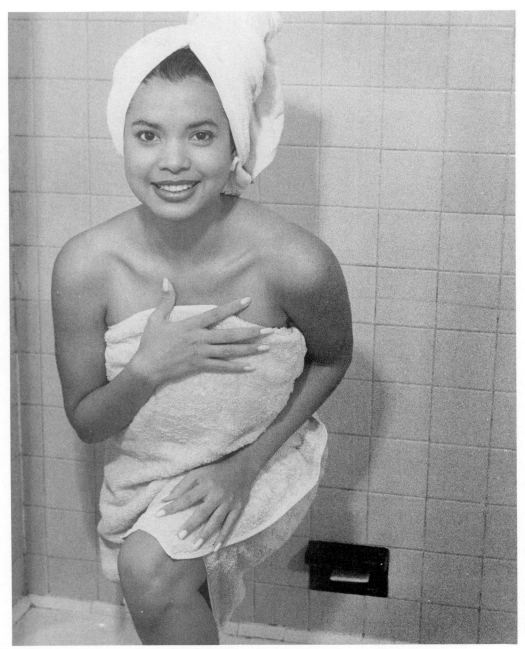

Use 100% cotton towels or towels made of natural fibers to dry and stimulate the skin after a bath.

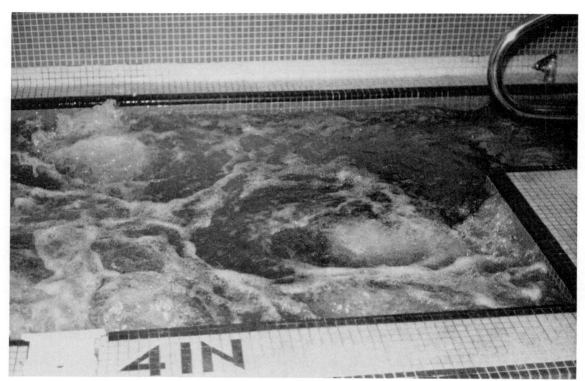

A whirlpool in action.

4
WHIRLPOOL BATHS AND HOT TUBS

Whirlpools are beautifully styled large or small bathtubs used for relaxation and for therapeutic and recreational purposes. They usually have jets that pump out water and cause it to move rapidly, creating a whirling effect. The water provides a soothing hydromassage, and can be anywhere from gently soothing to brisk and invigorating. Adjustable jets can be purchased so that you can assemble your own model. Whirlpools can contain as much as several hundred gallons of water and can be made from acrylic, fiberglass or even tile. Some whirlpools today even feature built-in hot and cold faucets, wood-grain floors and slip-resistant bottoms and come in many colors to fit your decor. Other accessories to heighten your experience in the whirlpool may include music, skylights, planters, video monitors and exercise machines.

The name Jacuzzi has become familiar in association with the whirlpool. Roy Jacuzzi is today chief executive officer of Jacuzzi Inc. The firm was established as the Jacuzzi Brothers by his grandfather and six brothers in 1915, when its main product was agricultural pumps. In 1968 Roy Jacuzzi produced and developed the Jacuzzi tub and it has since become a part of the family business. The first Jacuzzis were designed to provide a bigger space than the traditional bathtub, based on the ever-growing use of the house as a recreation and entertainment center. Some whirlpool baths will accommodate more than one person or a group of people. They can be found in homes, boats, spas, and even planes.

One whirlpool model available from Jacuzzi serves as both a bathtub and a spa. It is completely pre-plumbed and can be installed in the same way as a bathtub. A plumber simply hooks up the incoming hot and cold water lines to the water valve. The unit is self-enclosed, with a four-inch rim and can either be top-mounted or flush-mounted.

Some whirlpool baths are up to seven square feet and nearly thirty inches deep (this size will have nearly a 700-gallon capacity). A number of whirlpool companies will create a custom whirlpool bath upon request.

If you use a whirlpool at your health club or at a spa, look for signs of poor maintenance. Check the corners of the whirlpool for traces of foam or scum. This is an indication that the filtration system is inadequate. Since bacteria can thrive in the whirlpool's warm, recycled water, avoid using any facility that isn't spotlessly clean. Examine the edges to see if there is a dark line or ring. This is another sign of careless maintenance.

The combination of heat and rotating water makes whirlpool baths effective in many ways. What are some of the benefits?

helps sports injuries of all types

breaks up cellulite

increases circulation

helps varicose veins and sprains

relaxes and stretches tight, tense muscles

relieves bursitis, minor aches and pains

relaxes spasms

softens scar tissue

massages muscles

cleanses pores

dispels fatigue and rejuvenates

There is something almost indescribable about the energy of swiftly whirling water. It seems to be almost electric as it sends tiny surges of energy through the body. The whirlpool bath will allow your experience of pleasant sensations to be a healthy one also. Your body will be gently massaged and stimulated from head to toe, thus restoring tranquility and balance to your entire system. After a few minutes in the hot water, the body begins to relax and synchronize itself to the pulsating rhythm. This repetitive sensation harmonizes and organizes the body.

> For a sports injury where swelling may occur, put ice on the area immediately, and continue ice applications off and on for forty-eight hours. After two days (if you have a serious injury), start whirlpool treatments twice a day. The water temperature should be at least 100°F.

Cellulite and the whirlpool have a definite connection. As the trapped-in fat contained in cellulite receives the deep massage action of forced air and water, it loosens and begins to break up slightly. Just as deep-tissue massage may be helpful in displacing cellulite, the whirlpool may also provide some help.

Hot tubs, common in the Orient, were made popular in the U.S. during the back-to-nature movement of the 1960s and 1970s. Their wood frames and hot bubbling water created the perfect intimate environment for relaxed socializing and even business gatherings. However, because of the spread of AIDS, the hot tub is no longer as popular as the whirlpool.

Much deeper than the whirlpool bath, the hot tub allows the user to stand up and even walk around in it. Jet streams push the water around the tub, though there is much less of a whirling action than in whirlpool baths.

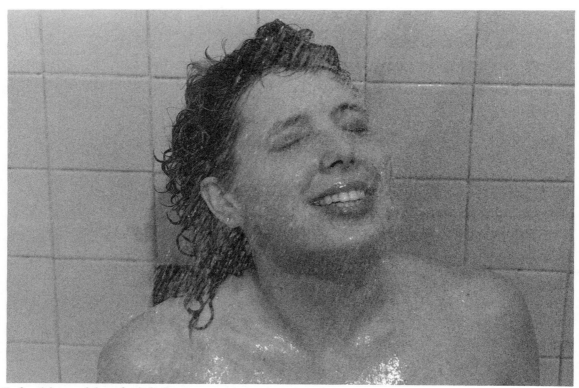

Refreshing with a facial shower.

5
SPRINKLE, SPRINKLE: THE BENEFITS OF A SHOWER

A shower is a downfall of water, usually from a source higher than the head. This downward movement of water generates energy and pressure as it trickles or pours down. The type of shower we are most familiar with is the bath shower, in which water is sprayed on the bather from an overhead nozzle. The nozzle allows the water to be dispersed over the body or localized in one small spot.

The therapeutic value of the shower is determined by the force or pressure of the water, the temperature of the water, the texture of the spray (hard or soft) and the area of the body in which it is used. The general effect is as follows:

- Gentle, quick, warm showers relax and harmonize
- Gentle, quick, cold showers stimulate and energize
- Short, cold showers stimulate

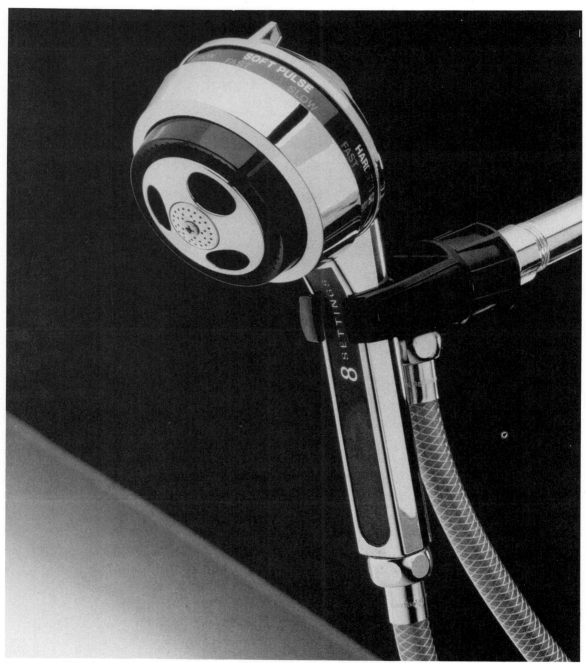

An example of a therapeutic showerhead with eight distinct shower settings.

- Long, cold showers relax
- Short, warm showers relax
- Long, warm showers energize and stimulate
- Jets or heavy streams relax but energize

Modern pressurized showerheads allow you to adjust the direction, volume and velocity of the oncoming water in an exciting blend of water techniques. A fine misty spray will gently caress your body, while a strong, focused jet will help relieve your aches and pains. Don't be afraid to experiment: Try shifting the spray to several different headings during the course of your shower.

Going from a gentle hot setting to one that is powerful and cold during one shower session will offer a boost to the circulatory system. This in turn may result in temporary relief from tension and high blood pressure.

Most special massage showerheads are easy to install. It usually involves removing the old showerhead with a wrench or pliers, then simply screwing the new one on over the existing threads. Often, if you are having trouble removing the old showerhead, a lubricating oil placed around the shower connection will help loosen it.

Actions of the shower are:

tonic for the entire body

reduces fever

restores vitality

cleanses the body

soothes tired muscles

stimulates circulation

relieves arthritic joints

soothes nerves

offers a place of solitude to hear yourself think

Showers, like other water treatments, can be applied in several different ways, depending primarily on the water temperature and area of the body being concentrated upon. Hot and cold showers serve different therapeutic purposes, as discussed below.

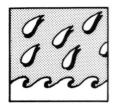

COLD SHOWERS

Cold water contracts the blood vessels if only a short cold shower is taken. It will no doubt recharge your batteries. If cold water is applied for long periods, it will have a different effect on the body, sedating and desensitizing it to pain.

The best way to enter the cold shower is a personal choice. If you are not the type to just jump in, start out with body-temperature water and gradually make it cooler until your body accepts the cold water.

When taking a short cold shower, remember that the water should be *really* cold. Stay under it for ten to twenty seconds; move out of it for the same length of time. Repeat the cycle at least three times, or as many times as you like.

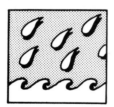

HOT SHOWERS

The main action of the hot shower is that it relaxes and enhances circulation. Again, the choice about entering it is up to you. However, with hot showers, it is best to begin with the water at body temperature and gradually increase it, because extremely hot water can damage your skin. When you are using the hot shower for its benefits to other parts of the body, use a cool compress on your forehead. This will prevent headaches and help balance the body heat. Applying the compress around the neck will achieve the same results.

To receive the full benefits of the hot shower, let the water build to the hottest possible temperature. Stay in the shower for thirty seconds to one minute (depending on your tolerance). Hot showers have a better cleansing penetration than do cold showers. The hot shower opens pores,

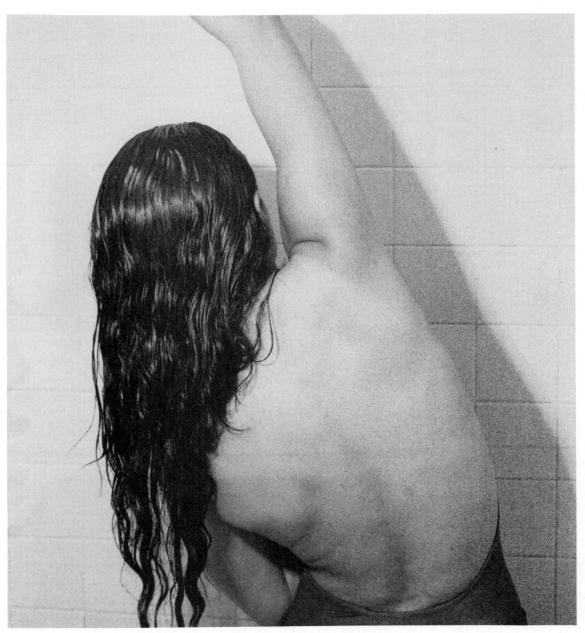

Abdominal Twist: Standing straight up, twist your entire body to the left. Hold the position for a few seconds, then twist your whole body to the right and hold for a few seconds. Repeat three times. This exercise will energize your whole body.

while cold showers close them. As the pores open, dead cells and other useless materials are ejected from the skin. In addition, the hot shower stimulates surface blood flow, which may result in a healthier, more vibrant skin tone.

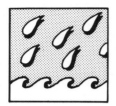

NEUTRAL SHOWERS

This is the most widely used shower. The neutral shower is made by turning on hot and cold water together until the temperature feels "just right." This type of shower has a characteristic all its own: Most important is the body's ability to stay in it for relatively long periods of time. Since it is comfortable, it creates a pleasurable environment. As the tepid water fills the tub, your body rises into a state of focus and equilibrium. That may seem like a small benefit, but it may well be one of the most important stress reducers available. A neutral shower provides the perfect place to spend a moment by yourself, completely alone and at peace. It is a place of pure sanctuary and calmness.

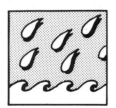

ALTERNATING HOT AND COLD SHOWERS

My favorite type of shower is the alternating hot and cold shower. As stated in the chapter on baths, the application of hot, then cold, water has a powerful effect on the system. While hot water opens pores, increases blood flow and puts all systems on go, cold applications close pores, slows blood flow and tells all systems to take a break. This type of shower is excellent to enhance poor circulation, muscular rheumatism, stiff joints, minor aches and pains and chronic backaches. In essence, it gives a boost to the entire system, promoting an overall feeling of well-being.

To use this technique, stay under the hot water for up to one minute, following it immediately with a cold jet spray for thirty seconds. Repeat the routine at least three times.

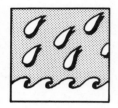

LOCALIZED SHOWERS

Localized showers are directed to one part of the body only, thus concentrating energy and blood flow in one specific area. As you may know by now, the object of healing is to increase blood flow in the desired area, which brings with it nutrients, natural pain relievers and rejuvenating properties.

Our bodies function as a complete unit, with each part bearing a connection to another part. Reflex points are places in the body that have a healing effect on another part of the body when they are stimulated. Localized showers will allow you to bring comfort to parts of your body that may be painful or tense by stimulating the reflex points in your feet and hands.

Keep in mind that our hands store excess tension and, in addition, house many reflex points. Thus, what a marvelous way to massage the entire body by simply localizing the shower spray on your hands. Alternate the spray on and off for at least five minutes. Hands should be flexible but strong, and you should not feel them tightening or cramping. I am sure you will enjoy the hand shower.

When spraying the feet, turn your soles upward and allow the spray to cover the entire foot. It is usually best to use heavy pressure on the feet, hands, back and neck, while a gentle spray is best on the forehead.

The abdominal shower will help relieve constipation and stomach discomforts. Simply direct the spray to the navel. The spray should be concentrated here for at least seven minutes, on and off, with thirty-second rest periods in between.

To increase breathing and counteract asthma, you will find that the chest shower has dramatic results, opening up the entire body. Alternate

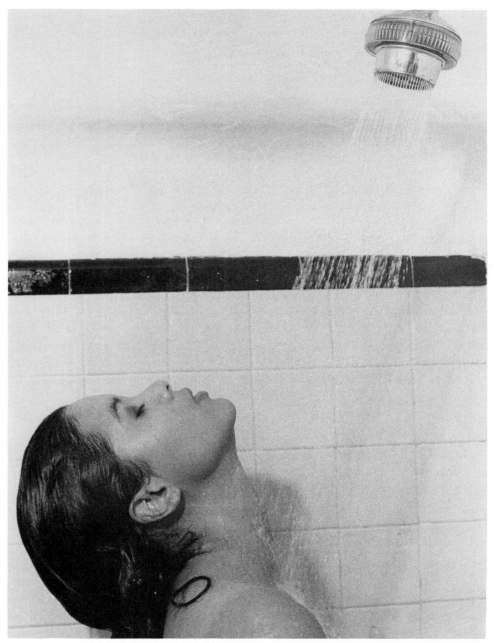

Localized shower (neck and throat): A marvelous way to relieve an irritated throat or stiff neck or both.

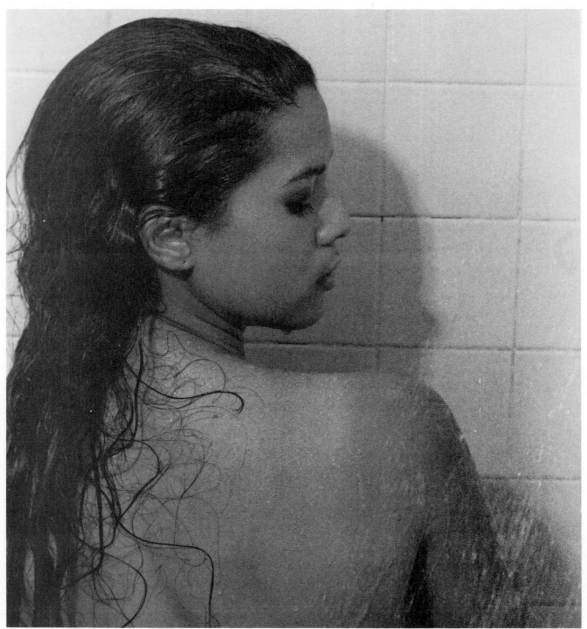

Localized shower (shoulder): Allow warm water to stay on the shoulder for three to five minutes. This relieves stiff shoulders and the day's tension while also increasing your circulation.

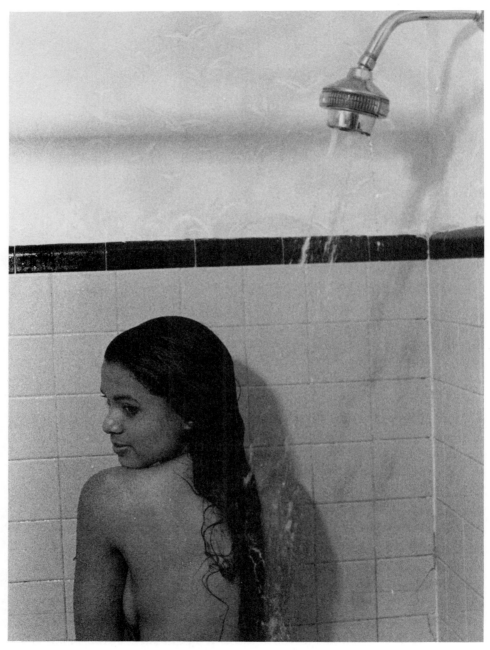

Localized shower (back): For a backache or tight muscles.

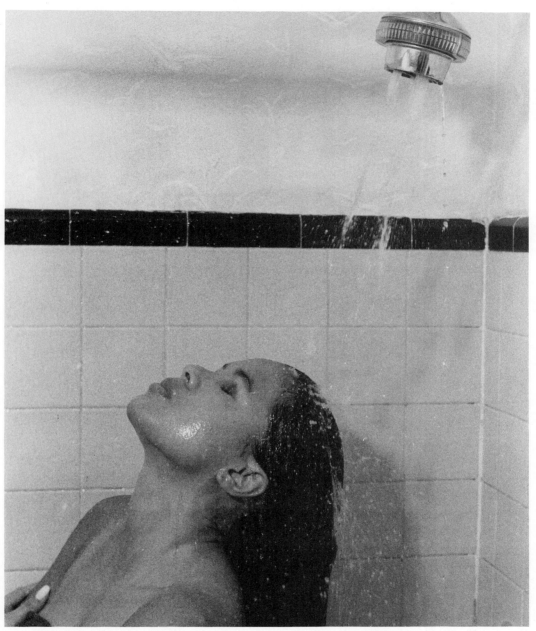

Localized shower (head): This type of shower can help relieve even the most persistent headache. It will also help enhance circulation for a glowing, more beautiful facial complexion.

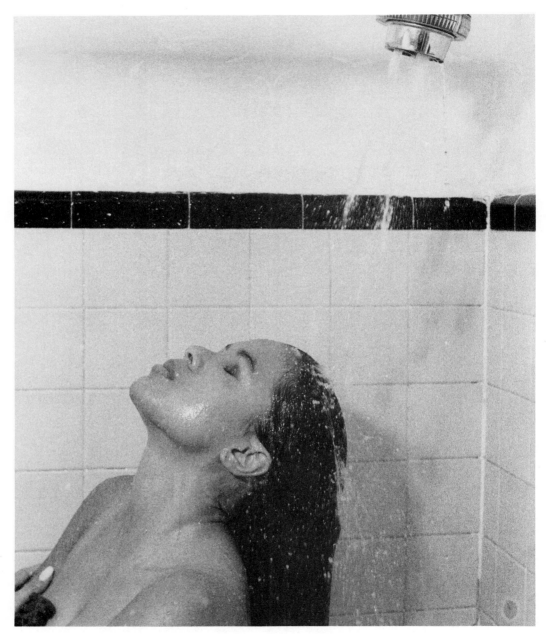

By standing under the shower with the water pulsating on your head, you can enhance the circulation throughout your entire body. You will feel relaxed and have a clearer state of mind.

the spray from light to heavy. (Heart patients are warned that this is a very powerful type of shower and may have an adverse action on the heart. Consult your physician before trying this.)

For those who use their voices a great deal and may develop an irritated throat, the neck shower is superb. Direct the jet at the center of your neck on all four sides. Hold your head back when applying water to the front and let it drop to the sides for side applications, finally dropping your head when spraying the back of your neck.

One extra benefit from the neck shower is that it helps your overall being. Not only does it carry with it physical benefits, but emotional ones as well. In fact, for persons who choke on their words and lack the confidence to speak their minds, the throat shower is strongly recommended.

When our energies are blocked, they do not flow properly and cause congestion in the body. This congestion will, for the most part, have a negative influence on our functioning. Perhaps Mother Nature has provided us with showers as an easy way of clearing channels of blocked energy. The emotional benefits of the shower are many. Perhaps you will discover even more as you apply it to your own health and beauty routine.

The Head Shower

The old-fashioned hair shampoo and rinse may have more benefits than you think. To stimulate the scalp, make a tea infusion by mixing two tablespoons of rosemary, sage or peppermint tea with three cups of boiling water. Turn the flame off and allow the tea to steep for at least fifteen minutes. Strain the herbs so only the liquid rinse remains. Wet your hair with warm water and slowly massage the rinse into your scalp. Let it remain while you shower the rest of your body. After five minutes or so, rinse it out with cool water. Massage your scalp vigorously as you do this. This rinse is known to have powerful rejuvenating qualities for your brain, and increases hair growth. It also helps restore pH balance to your hair and scalp.

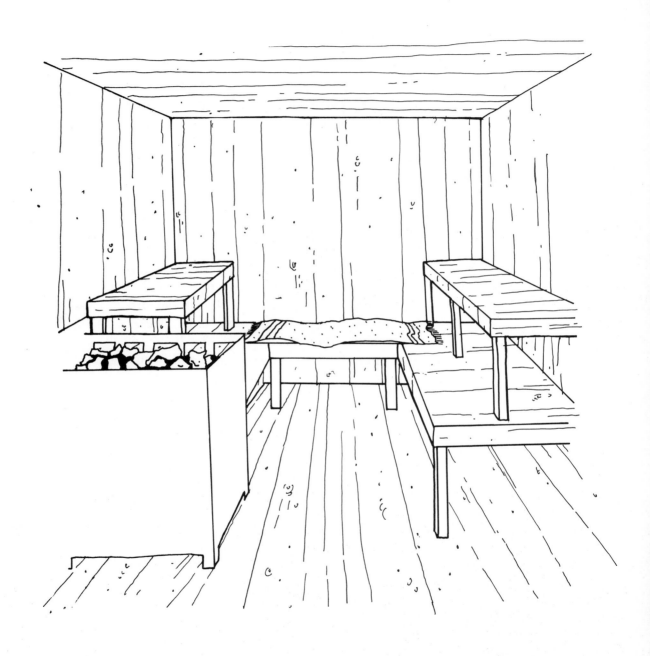

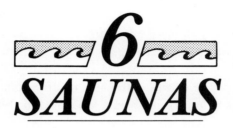

SAUNAS

Sauna is the Finnish word for an insulated wood-lined room, large or small, that is heated by a special stove. The stove contains stones and is erected specifically to create the environment for a dry-heat bath. The object is to make you sweat. The more you sweat, the better. By inducing perspiration, the sauna bath cleanses the skin and stimulates internal circulation. It is also used purely for relaxation. The sauna experience can be described as a rejuvenating and rebirthing of the mind and body. It is a total experience, benefiting every system and part of the body.

The actions of a sauna bath are so numerous it would take an entire book to list and explain each one. However, here are a few:

energizes

relaxes muscle spasms

relieves arthritic pain

eliminates toxins

stimulates hair growth

fosters weight loss

opens blocked respiratory passages

cleanses skin and opens pores

increases circulation

relieves stress and anxiety

combats fatigue

acts as a refresher

Prolonged use and overuse of the sauna should be avoided, as there may be reverse effects due to exposure to too much dry heat too frequently. Three to four saunas a week—for a maximum of fifteen minutes each—will allow the body a chance to readjust in between saunas.

A forerunner of the sauna is the sun itself, which provides dry heat. Roman bathhouses of antiquity had a steam room heated with a special boiler. Like Russian, Turkish and Egyptian bathhouses, they were places for social gathering and philosophical conversation. The Irish used sweating houses made of stone, and in Germany water was poured over hot stones to produce steam as bathers brushed each other with medicinal branches.

So-called sweat lodges are found throughout history, from Africa to America. A sweat lodge is a tepee- or house-like structure made of heavy cloths. Hot rocks are placed within, in a central pit. Bathers stay in it until they sweat profusely. They use natural cloth materials to rub their skin while they sweat.

Sweat pits had a major role in the lives of native Americans, who used them for physical, emotional, spiritual and ceremonial purposes. Groups would gather inside to pray, chant, sing or simply relax together. The sweat pit was actually a conical hut, about one and a half meters high, set partly in the ground and made of packed earth. The opening was covered by a removable cloth; several large stones were heated on an open fire outside, and when they were hot enough, they were shoveled into the pit. Eskimos also use the sweat hut.

Native Americans took great care with sweat lodge construction. Whenever possible, the lodges were built near cool water, as users periodically left the tent for cold dips. Often four or five cycles of sweating and cooling off were used in alternative fashion to complete one sweat session.

There were often separate huts for different purposes. Much the same way a boxer conjures up his energy through working up a sweat before a fight, Indian men thought power and vitality would come to them from sweating. In addition, certain firewoods were burned in the huts because of their aromatic or purported medicinal qualities.

The inhabitants of Finland have known about and used saunas for over two thousand years. Like the American Indians, they believe that the intense heat and fire elements present in the sauna have an almost divine power. Nature provided their land with abundant timber and proper stones for the building and optimal usage of the sauna. In earlier times, Finnish women often went into the sauna to give birth, and farmers found the sauna a useful place to dry out their farm produce.

There are more than one million saunas in Finland today. Nearly one out of every four households has a sauna. In fact, whenever a new home is built, the construction of a sauna is routinely considered. Most hotels and health facilities, including hospitals, also have them. Nor are commercial and private saunas strangers to the U.S. They present a cost-effective, safe and efficient way to achieve and maintain good health.

Saunas may be heated by smoke sauna stoves or heat storage stoves (wood, gas, oil, electric). The typical sauna is a single room housed in a log structure set among trees in wooded areas or on the shores of a lake. These natural vistas provide an environment of tranquility and peace that can be enjoyed before and after the sauna. Large saunas sometimes even include a dining room and lounging deck; or, they can be conveniently located to provide access to supporting units, such as dressing rooms, stove rooms and washrooms.

A *vihta* or a *brisk* is a broad bundle of leafy birch twigs, cut during late spring and summer. Birch and other leaves, such as eucalyptus or oak, can also be used (all have healing properties). The *brisk* is usually twenty to twenty-four inches long and is stored in a cool place when not in use. The loofah sponge can also be used during a sauna bath by rubbing the body briskly to stimulate the skin and enhance circulation.

When the sauna is operating, heat rises roughly 10° for every one foot above the floor level. Thus, when you are sitting in the sauna, your head is the hottest and your feet are the coolest. When you lie down, the reverse happens. This position brings benefits of its own: It will greatly aid circulation throughout the body and soothe tired feet. Place your feet in a raised position by resting them on a rolled towel or stool. In the sauna, the drier the heat, the more one can tolerate it. The temperature at head height should be at least 158°F. Thermometers should be hung at head level for easy viewing.

In a properly heated sauna, perspiration will occur sufficiently. The stones should be so hot that water thrown on them will immediately produce steam. They should also be insulated by covering them on both sides with a frame to reduce direct radiation of heat in the room; the heat should instead be dispersed in all directions. Saunas built of rough wood, without varnish or oils, are the best type. The benches should be smooth and comfortable, and there should also be footrests. The overall design should be simple and tranquil, with subtle and subdued lighting. Natural oils will enhance the aromatic atmosphere; wood scents such as pine, wintergreen or sandalwood make good selections. Water can be added to the hot rocks to produce a vapor, with purifying effects.

A considerable amount of research has been done on the physiological effects of saunas. Of these, a rise in body temperature and perspiration are the most significant. Skin temperatures may rise to 104°F in less than five minutes. The body reacts to the intense heat by releasing perspiration, which then cools the skin as it evaporates. Surface blood vessels become enlarged. This brings an increased amount of blood flow to the surface as skin cells receive increased nourishment. Heat is then transferred to the deeper parts of the body. The water from perspiration offers relief to the kidneys. Toxins are released through oxidation, which is increased due to the intense heat.

Used to clear acne and skin problems, dry heat is excellent. The pores open and unclog skin cells. Blood flow is increased as the skin is fed by blood that comes from the heart's pumping. High blood pressure drops temporarily because of the dilation of the blood vessels. There is reason to believe that persons who use sauna over a period of time, and with regularity, have blood vessels that remain elastic and pliable longer because of the healthy dilation and contraction. In fact, all organs, muscles and tissues are stimulated when sauna is used. Note, however, that **persons with heart defects, circulatory disorders, skin ailments or similar health conditions should consult a physician before using the sauna.**

The sore muscles and stiff limbs and joints that frequently follow sports participation are helped by the sauna bath. Through free perspiration, sauna helps disperse excess lactic acid built up and stored in the muscles. This is especially true after strenuous exercising or workouts. The considerable amount of water lost through the sauna process (this can be as much as a half-gallon of water) can result in temporary weight loss and regulation of kidney function. It must be remembered, however, that whenever profuse perspiration occurs, water should be drunk to replace valuable minerals that are also lost.

From sweating out a cold to resting frazzled nerves, the environment of the sauna is healing. Sauna penetrates into the subcutaneous tissue, invigorating the muscles and joints and directly affecting ailing connective tissue with powerful healing results. One byproduct is an improvement in skin tone. Salt is removed from the skin through perspiration, and this may have positive effects in lowering high blood pressure. (Researchers have discovered that heart patients may benefit by the body's release of excess sodium.)

The system most affected by the sauna is the circulatory system. While the body temperature increases, the brain is alerted and commands a series of actions. Body metabolism speeds up as we sweat in order to cool off. During a sauna bath, most water is lost primarily through the skin on the forehead, neck and trunk. Feet and hands may or may not sweat in the sauna; they respond to emotional stimuli and not generally to heat or exercise.

The following is a recommended sauna routine:

two minutes warm shower

ten minutes sauna

two minutes cold plunge, swim, cold shower or brief rest

ten minutes sauna

two minutes cold plunge, swim, cold shower or brief rest

ten minutes sauna

cool shower

The alternating hot-and-cold sequences produce an exhilarating feeling. (Again, heart patients check with your physician first!)

In ancient Egypt, it was believed that drops of perspiration allegedly from the body of the god Osiris had sacramental value.

Here are some general health rules for the sauna user:

• Move back and forth, from the top to the bottom bench
• Never enter the sauna after taking medication

- Don't overdo it. At the first sign of discomfort, dizziness or shortness of breath, it's time to take a break
- Eat one hour before and one hour after entering the sauna
- Remove all clothing, except possibly a thin cotton towel
- Try light exercise, meditation or even prayer in the sauna
- Use a natural brush or loofah for rubbing the skin during and after the sauna
- Alternate with a cool dip in shower, pool or lake

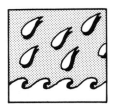

A FACIAL MASSAGE IN THE SAUNA

Here is a good facial massage technique to use while in the shower after a sauna. It will help firm and tone your skin.

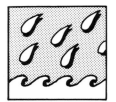

A HOT OIL HAIR TREATMENT IN THE SAUNA

The sauna is also the perfect place to give your hair an invigorating hot oil hair treatment. Hot oil treatments may be of considerable help in repairing split ends and stimulating hair growth. Choose a natural conditioner such as rosemary or tea and follow this recipe: Boil three cups of water. Place two tablespoons of rosemary or tea in the water, turn off the flame and let the mixture steep for a half hour. Pour off the rosemary or tea for the rinse. Add three tablespoons of olive oil to the remaining liquid and massage into your scalp just before entering the sauna. Cover your head with a swimming or shower cap (cotton cloth is best). Sit in the sauna for ten minutes, take a break and reenter for another five minutes. Wash the rinse out with warm water. After the entire process, massage your head in a brisk, circular movement, using your fingertips. Drink a large glass of water to finish.

The sauna is a place of release, purge and cathartic experience, a place to cleanse and rejuvenate. If you have not done so already, make plans to kick back, take it nice and slow, heat it up and let your energies flow . . . in the sauna!

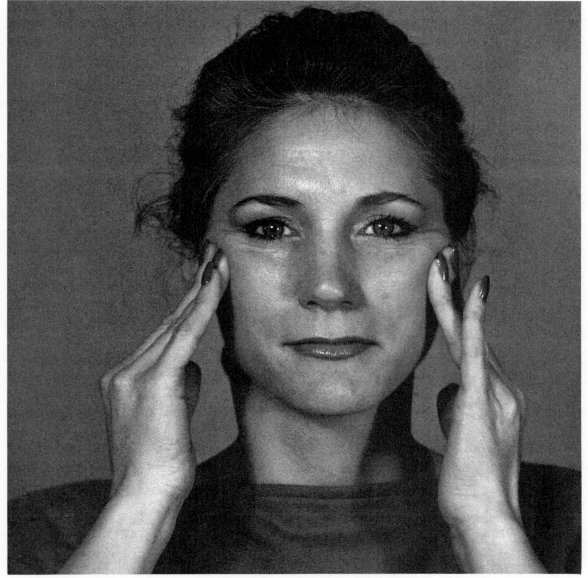

Esthetic massage for the face. Rotate in small circles while lifting gently toward the eyes.

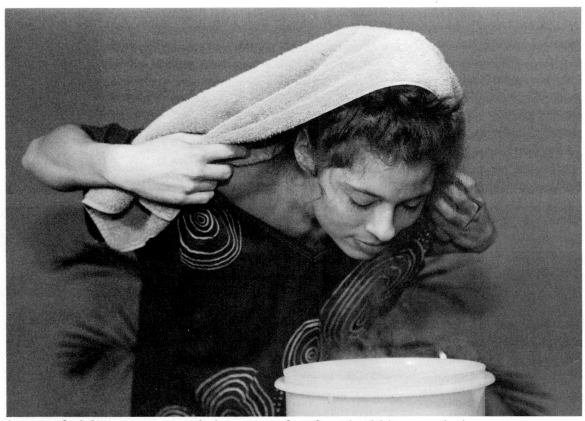

A steam facial opens pores and cleans your face for a healthier complexion.

7
STEAM BATHS

We move now from the dry heat of the sauna to the moist or wet heat of the steam bath. Steam is the gaseous vapor state of water. It is actually the mist of cooling water vapor, and is produced by heating water to a high temperature. The wet heat of steam is valuable in stimulating every part of the body. Most of all, steam has a deep, penetrating action that eases itself into the pores and underlying skin tissues. It causes an increase in skin temperature, which in turn allows the body to emit perspiration, thereby carrying toxins out of the body.

There are many forms in which steam can be applied. The most common are the full-body treatment available in a steam bath—an enclosed room in which steam is forced out through pipes and fills the room; and the facial treatment—usually the steam is generated from boiling water, or from commercial facial steamers.

The actions of a steam bath are:

opens pores

opens clogged nostrils

increases respiration

helps relieve bronchitis

cleanses the body

offers relief for sore and irritated throat

increases circulation

helps relieve asthma

opens sinuses

refreshens and enlivens

tones muscles and joints

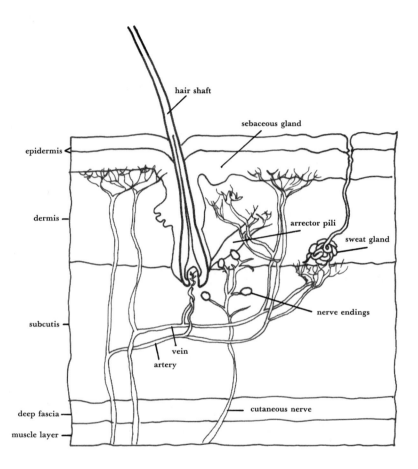

epidermis

dermis

subcutis

deep fascia

muscle layer

hair shaft

sebaceous gland

arrector pili

sweat gland

nerve endings

vein

artery

cutaneous nerve

A skin cell. Steaming and other forms of hydrotherapy stimulate cellular skin glands.

Vaporizers are a convenient method for emitting steam into the air. The action of steam in your home may help to neutralize the air and add moisture to it, especially in the winter and summer, when over-heating and air-conditioning dry out the air. As moisture is added to the air, the room is cleansed as harmful pollutants are dissolved and evaporated.

Moist air has long been known for its healing benefits. When distilled water is used in vaporizers or humidifiers, it has very much the same effect in the air as it does when you drink it. Since distilled water is void of all minerals and solids, it will absorb substances it comes in contact with. For this reason, distilled water is the best type to use when you are seeking a purifying or cleansing effect. Mineral or spring water will also have a beneficial effect on the body. When used in a vaporizer or humidifier, it will add minerals and other health-giving substances to the air that your body can then inhale and digest. Certain herbs and other natural substances are useful as inhalants to increase respiration by opening breathing passages. Serious chest problems resulting from bronchial complications find relief with warm, moist heat that is produced by steam. Actually, steam is an ingenious gift of nature when you think about it: The combination of water and heat, packaged into a soothing, natural form, is useful to athletes, health seekers and beauty lovers alike. Best of all, this wonderful element can be used in perfect harmony with other water therapies, such as saunas, ice treatments or baths.

In your own home, you can use steam by hot water to penetrate tired and aching muscles, ease arthritis and lower back pain and help heal fractures and sprains. Simply aim the steam from a spouted teapot in the direction of the specific area and allow the steam to saturate it.

Steam rooms are usually regulated by the use of a thermostat that cuts off steam when it goes beyond a certain temperature. This feature allows you to soak up as much steam as you need in one sitting, with breathers in between as the room automatically cools off. While using the steam room, it is beneficial to gently stretch out tight muscles as your body settles into the steam. Try to stay in the steam room for at least five minutes. Leave, take a cold shower for two to three minutes and return for another five minutes. Leave and once again shower in cool or cold water. This routine can be repeated until you feel satisfied that you have completed the cycle. To measure the steam bath's effectiveness, taste the perspiration on your skin. If it has a very salty taste, you may want to repeat another cycle. When it no longer tastes salty, you have had enough. Always drink a glass of fresh water afterward to replace the valuable minerals lost during perspiration.

In the steam room, an almost reverent attitude is gradually felt by most of the participants. They sit receptively, waiting for the comforting bursts of hot, wet vapor that will soon cause them to exit quickly, saturated from head to toe with perspiration. It is best to take a cool shower immediately before and after using the steam for optimal benefits. At my health club, a combination of natural oils such as peppermint, wintergreen or eucalyptus is used as inhalants in the steam room, always giving it the aroma of the fresh outdoors.

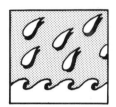 ## A BEAUTY FACIAL USING STEAM

Facial steam baths make it possible for you to beautify your face in several easy steps. All you need are the following items:

- small saucepan
- one quart of water
- three tablespoons of any of the following: rosemary, peppermint, or camomile
- small mixing bowl
- full-size bath towel

Boil the water in the saucepan. Put the herb or oil in the bowl and pour the boiling water over it. Immediately, place your head over the bowl, with the towel covering your face and head, creating a tentlike effect.

As an alternative, several companies make facial steamers that are designed for this purpose. The Herbal Sauna by Aunu is available by mail and is the best commercial facial steamer available. Its blend of natural herbs, oils and other ingredients soothe, soften and nourish the skin, while also increasing facial circulation. In addition, its aroma is very pleasing. (To order Aunu products, see page 146.)

8
ENEMAS AND COLONICS

The main purpose of an enema is to release recently gathered matter from the stomach. This matter consists of waste materials and poisons that may only be reached by purging of the colon. An enema cleans the lower colon. The main purpose of a colonic, by contrast, is to clean the entire colon. Both enemas and colonics stimulate the kidneys and liver and stomach action. They also help to reduce pelvic pain and give a boost to the functioning of the entire digestive system. The feeling afterward is one of cleanliness and inner release.

Most adults have pounds of toxic matter stored in the colon that eventually causes skin eruptions, a tired and sluggish feeling, overweight, nervousness and low stress levels. Eventually, cancer and high blood pressure may also be the result of internal impurities. An entire book could be written about the importance of a clean colon. It probably is the single most important factor in maintaining a healthy and beautiful body. Foods that are difficult to digest—red meat, dairy, fried foods—may not assimilate properly into the body and thus are eliminated as useless. Unfortunately, this matter does not pass through the colon, but remains there, sometimes for years and years. Drinking fresh-squeezed juices and plenty of water and eliminating excessive fried foods, dairy and red meat from your diet will insure the good health of your colon.

Colonics are more thorough than enemas. However, unlike enemas, which can be self-administered in your own home, they require that you find a trained professional who has both a caring attitude and sterile equipment. Many nurses are trained in administering colonics; consult your local telephone directory for practitioners. **Always check with your physician before taking a colonic, as some conditions are contraindicated for colonics.** These include colitis, yeast infections, diverticulitis, advanced pregnancy and cancer.

Colonic therapists often will guide you through a relaxing visualization during the session, which is geared not only to cleansing the body but also to releasing pent-up emotions such as anger and fear (there is a direct relationship between negative emotions and a blocked colon).

Taking an enema is easy to do: Obtain an enema bag from your local drugstore and fill it with warm water (you may add an infusion of peppermint tea, finely strained, or two tablespoons of fresh lemon juice). There are two positions you can use. In the first, lie flat on your side and insert the nozzle from the rear. In the second, hang the enema bag overhead so the water trickles down. Rest on all fours, tilt your upper body down toward the floor and insert the nozzle from this position. At first, allow a small amount of water in, stop the flow and relax. You will feel pressure when the anal cavity is full. Hold the water in as long as you can, then release it. You may take up to two bags of water in one session.

It is important to relax the entire time you take the enema. Be sure to let your breath flow, slowly inhaling and exhaling. A constricted breathing pattern will tighten the anal muscles, preventing the enema from working.

It is essential that enemas and colonics be taken during prolonged cleansing fasts. If not, the toxins released will back up in the system, causing a type of self-poisoning. During fasting, two enemas daily are recommended—one in the morning and another at night. Do not make enemas or colonics a way of life, however. There is a larger, easier and more foolproof method for cleaning out your internal body. The formula is simple: pure foods, exercise, positive thoughts and plenty of fresh, pure water.

To summarize: Waste material is accumulated in the tissues for years, causing disease and premature aging. These wastes can be eliminated from the system only by way of the kidneys, bowels, skin, and lungs. The alimentary canal, the bowels, is the main route by which these toxins are released from the body. When bowel movements cease to take place, toxic wastes have no way of leaving the system except with the help of enemas and colonics. To prevent toxins from reabsorbing into the system, it is therefore essential to cleanse the system. Otherwise your body will attempt to get the toxins out through other eliminative organs, particularly the kidneys, which will often be overloaded and even damaged as a result. Colonics and enemas assist the body in its cleansing and detoxifying effort by washing out all the toxic wastes from the alimentary canal.

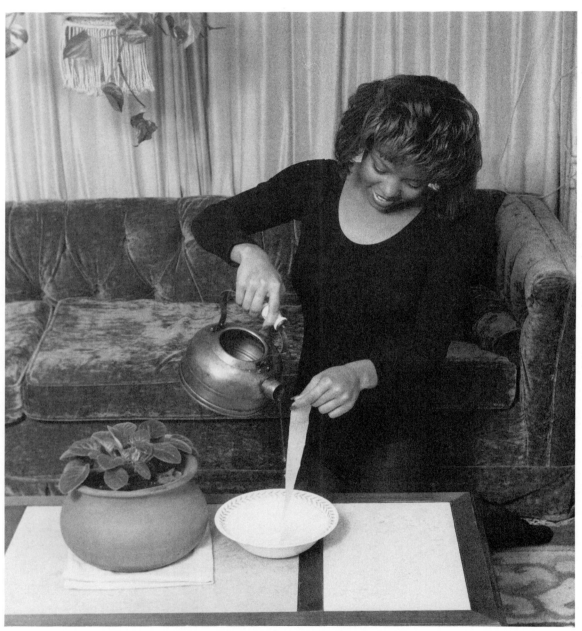

Making a hot compress: Boil water, then place thin cotton gauze or cloth into a bowl. Pour boiled water into the bowl and allow it to stand so that it cools enough so it will not burn but is still quite warm.

9
COMPRESSES
AND PACKS

A compress consists of folds of some soft material that is moistened and applied to a specific area of the body for therapeutic benefits. It may be left on for anywhere from five to fifteen minutes, depending on the purpose. Cold or hot water, herbs and essential oils may all be applied through the compress. These valuable healing elements come into direct contact with the body. Wintergreen or peppermint oil, for example, will both penetrate into the deeper tissues. There are some ready-made creams or oils on the market that can be used with compresses. Make sure, however, that they are as free as possible of synthetic and toxic ingredients before you use them.

There are three basic kinds of compresses: cold, hot and alternating hot and cold. Any or all can be used as herbal or medicated compresses as well.

Actions of the compress are:

relieves pain
removes stiffness in joints
improves tone and circulation
relieves spasms
helps mend and support bones
repairs and softens skin tissues
relieves pressure in sprains

stimulates sweat glands
stimulates lymphatic system
reduces swelling
helps rheumatic complaints
cleanses cuts and pimples
stimulates hair growth
diminishes headaches

Today, because it is possible to buy prepackaged herb teas, soothing relief is close at hand. For tired eyes, for example, apply a warm peppermint tea bag over your eyes while you relax.

Compresses can be applied anywhere on your body. Any ache, pain, discomfort or place of tension is waiting for the soothing, healing application of a compress. Once you know the effects of hot versus cold compresses, you will be able to aid in your own healing process, using this easy natural technique. And remember: Always seal and wrap the compress airtight, as the pressure resulting from the compress is in itself a beneficial element.

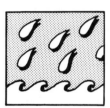

HOT COMPRESSES

To make a hot compress, boil water and try to keep it hot enough to reuse when the first compress cools. Prepare several cloths: Fold each cloth into thirds so that they retain surface heat. Dip the first cloth into the water, leaving the ends out of the water for easy handling. Wring out the center of the cloth. If you are using essential oil, or some other medication that is not already in the boiling water, this is the time to add it to the cloth. Apply the compress as soon as possible. The object is to build up as much heat on the skin surface as possible without letting it escape.

Keep in mind that the compress you make may be any size. It can be small enough to cover only a finger, or large enough to cover the entire chest. It is a good idea to test the skin with a small portion of the compress before applying the entire compress so that it does not burn the skin surface. If, in fact, it is too hot to apply in one motion, apply it a bit at a time, moving the cloth back and forth until the entire area is covered. Then, cover the first cloth with a dry cloth to seal in the heat and herbal vapors.

You should keep a compress on until it loses its heat and have another already prepared and ready to place on the area as soon as you remove the first (the longer the time in between applications, the weaker the results). It may be necessary to use at least three applications for most situations. After the final application, immediately run cold water over the body part for about two minutes or place a cool cloth over it.

For stomach or abdominal discomfort, place a large, hot compress on the stomach area. Then cover it with a flannel or woolen cloth to hold in the heat. Leave it on until it cools. Repeat with a second compress, remembering to cover it. Run cold water over stomach afterwards.

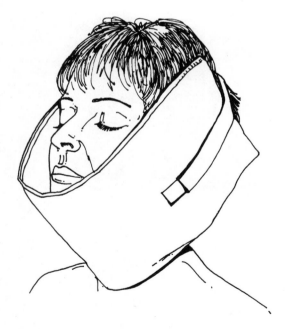

The Thermophore ™ **from Battle Creek is a moist-heat pack designed for the neck, throat, shoulder and other sinus areas. It produces its own moisture.**

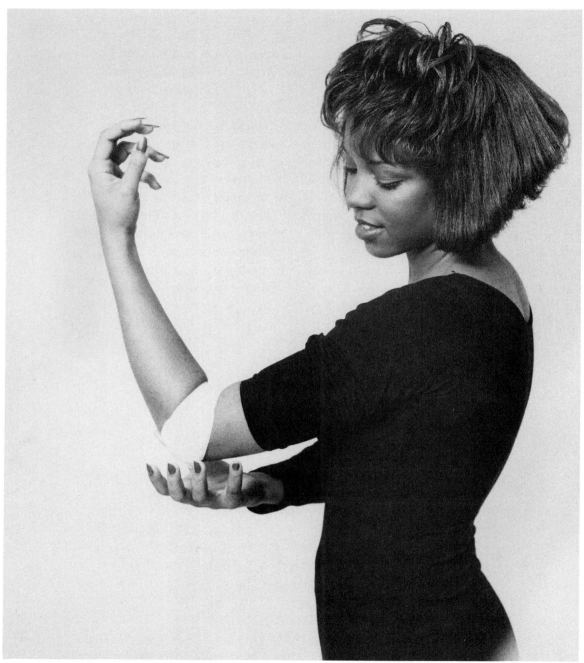

A compress on the elbow can help with tennis elbow and also facilitates circulation.

For enhancing the voice, and relieving neck stiffness, apply a hot compress around the entire neck. Fasten it with a safety pin or a clip to hold it tightly in place. Cover the compress with a woolen or flannel cloth. You can use a peppermint, eucalyptus or sage tea infusion as a soak on the compress.

Natural fibers (cotton, linen, wool) offer the best therapeutic value as compresses since the fibers breathe along with your skin and provide a greater penetration and absorbent quality.

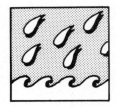 ## COLD COMPRESSES

The cold compress will constrict blood flow if it is applied for short periods of time (cold makes things grow smaller and more dense; heat expands them). For this reason, cold compresses are used primarily to relieve headaches and reduce swelling. Their other actions include:

reducing inflammation
relieving pain and muscular discomfort
preventing and reducing fever
soothing an irritated throat
rejuvenating skin tissues

To make a cold compress, fold a cotton or linen cloth into thirds and place it in ice water. Wring out the cloth and apply it to the desired area. When it begins to get lukewarm, replace it with another that has just been removed from the ice water. The object is to allow the skin surface a chance to get as cold as possible. However, when the area is a sensitive one, such as the face, be careful not to keep the cold compress on to the point of pain, as you may damage the tender cells in the facial skin. Usually, common sense will tell you when it's time to stop the applications. The colder the application, the shorter the time it needs to stay on. The duration can vary from ten to forty minutes.

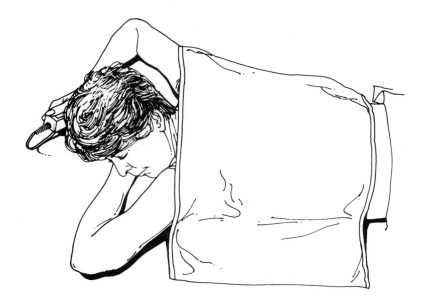

This large compress from Battle Creek is designed for use on the back, shoulder or knee. It too produces its own moisture.

Comfrey, an herb that has remarkable properties, is recommended whenever you want to use a cold compress that soothes, heals and nourishes. Prepare a tea infusion and when it cools off add it to ice water. The compress is then soaked in the infusion.

For a chest compress that helps break up congestion, relieve the effects of bronchitis and asthma and open up breathing passages, try the following: First, dip a medium-size bath towel into cold water. Wring out the towel until it is dripping slightly. Apply it to the chest. Cover it with a larger dry towel. Replace the wet towel in a few minutes, or add pieces of ice to it to maintain its coldness. Do this two or three times. When you complete the last application, rub the chest area briskly from top to bottom.

The use of compresses as a cosmetic aid will find you using one of my favorite beauty treatments. The purpose of this ten-minute session is to prevent excess oil from building up in the face, reduce acne and soften and cleanse your skin. It is an exquisite method for adding that special something to the appearance of your skin. You will need five items: water, a cotton washcloth, witch hazel, small cotton squares and a cucumber.

The treatment is in four easy steps. First, wash your face in warm water. Next, soak the cotton squares in witch hazel and place them all over your face. After they have been on for five to ten minutes, place a thin slice of cucumber over each eye. Peel the remainder of the cucumber. Squeeze or juice the cucumber and place it in a bowl of water. Soak more cotton squares in the cucumber water. Apply them to your face and let stand for five to ten minutes. Remove and rinse your face with cool water. At the end of this, you will feel an immediate difference. It is great as an instant pick-me-up and rejuvenator for your face.

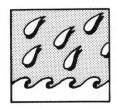 ## PACKS

The application of hot or cold packs over a compress may increase its effectiveness. A pack usually consists of several layers of natural fiber cloth, with ice or heat in between the layers. By layering the ice or heat in between cotton cloths, the valuable temperature is kept between the skin and the cloth, making the chosen treatment more effective as the skin gradually absorbs the benefits of the compress. In addition, the layered cloth provides protection for the skin from direct contact with the substance, whether it be ice or heat.

Other substances, such as clay, may also be used for packs; these are made into a paste and applied directly to the skin. Total body wraps are made by wrapping the person up in a sheet that has any of the therapeutic qualities of heat or cold. Facial packs are common, as is a simple folded cloth filled with crushed ice and applied to a sore or swollen part of the body.

The pack is an ancient and potent form of water therapy. Its actions are:

reduces fever
allays nervousness and tension

alleviates skin problems

relieves and mends joint stiffness

acts as a powerful external cleanser

relieves muscular pain

tones and rejuvenates

Here is a recipe for a total body pack that will draw toxins from your skin, leaving it refreshed and clean: Drink a cup of hot peppermint, sage or rosemary tea. Plunge a large white cotton sheet into hot water. Wring it out so that it remains damp and not soaking wet. Next, wrap the sheet around your entire body (your feet may be covered by cotton socks). Lie down on a woolen blanket. Make sure the wrap is secure and airtight. Stay wrapped in the sheet for at least fifteen minutes. After you remove the sheet, take a warm shower, brushing your body vigorously.

Mustard Packs

Mustard is a natural stimulant. The mustard pack has proved to be the friend of many tired muscles, offering them a soothing experience. The actions of the mustard pack include:

lowers blood pressure

relieves joint and muscle pain

relieves arthritis

increases circulation

improves muscle tone

breaks up internal congestion

relieves lower back pain

quickly heats the body

To make a mustard pack, fold a cotton or linen cloth into thirds. In a bowl, mix one tablespoon of dry mustard powder (found in most health-food stores) with four to eight tablespoons of flour. Moisten with warm water until well blended. Place the mixture inside the folded cloth. If you have a food steamer, place the cloth over the steamer to keep it hot. Lightly coat the skin over the desired area with olive or vegetable oil. Place the mustard pack over or around the area, cover it with a dry cloth and let it remain for at least ten minutes.

Earth Packs

The earth pack certainly ranks at the top of the list when it comes to water therapies that are also enjoyable. The fun of putting on a facial mask combines with an age-old remedy for preventing premature aging

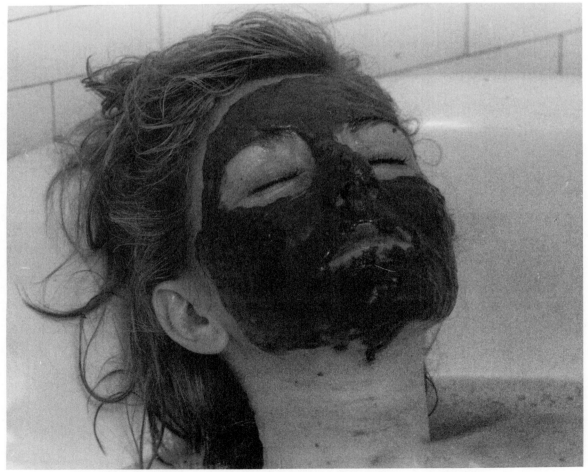

Deep-cleansing the facial skin with a clay facial mask can be very relaxing.

in the face through the use of hot sand, mud, clay or food. Common foods such as oatmeal, yogurt and honey are substances right at your fingertips that form the basis for useful packs. Deep-cleansing masks, made from green clay or various mineral muds, are available through most pharmacies or health-food stores.

The action of earth packs includes:

removes dead cells from skin surface
smooths and firms skin tissues

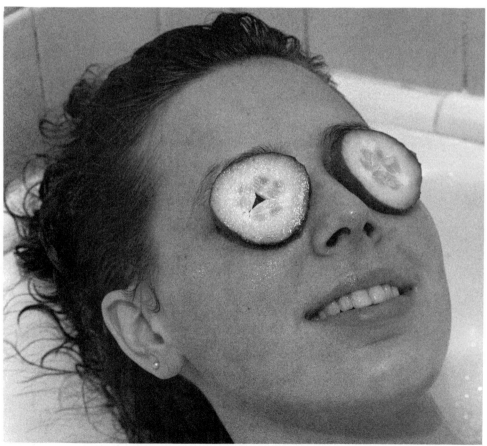

Cut two thin slices of cucumber, close your eyes and place one slice over each eye. Leave them on as long as three minutes. This is a real treat for tired eyes.

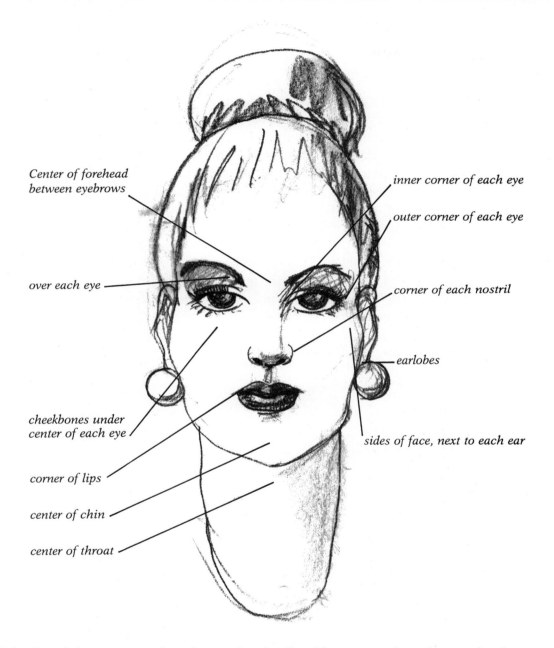

Center of forehead
between eyebrows

inner corner of *each eye*

outer corner of *each eye*

over each eye

corner of *each nostril*

earlobes

cheekbones under
center of each eye

sides of face, next to each ear

corner of lips

center of chin

center of throat

Before applying a mustard pack, try the simple self-massage of gently pressing in the direction of the arrows in the diagram above. This will make using the pack all the more relaxing. Drawing by Fred Bush.

relieves arthritis
relieves muscle spasms
nourishes skin

To make a facial pack, put two teaspoons of uncooked oatmeal and ten to fifteen tablespoons of plain sugar-free yogurt in the blender and mix. Place the mixture on your face, working from the neck to the top of your forehead. Be sure to cover the back of your neck and behind your ears. Leave it on your face for ten to fifteen minutes, then wash off with warm water. Your face will be the recipient of nourishing, soothing and cleansing properties that will leave it with a good feeling.

Once again, if you purchase herbs or other substances for your face and body, make absolutely sure that you only use the best quality and purest form for the best results. If you are not able to find green or white clays, write to Aphrodisia Herbs at 282 Bleecker Street, New York, N.Y. 10014 (212-989-6440). There are many different combinations that you can blend together to create healing and health-giving packs. If you've mastered the basic packs, begin to experiment: Try adding your favorite fragrance to them, or even add natural ingredients to enhance the colors.

10
ICE: A REMEDY FOR ACHES AND PAINS

The freezing point of water is 32°F (0°C). If the water is mixed with other substances, or is impure in any other way, the freezing point may be lower.

Ice has the power to heal, soothe and beautify. It is easy to make and one of the best natural therapies available. Ice is a natural anesthetic, chilling the senses until nerve endings become numb or desensitized. For this reason, it can help reduce the discomfort of strains, aches, pains and sprains. Used as an astringent, it tightens and beautifies the skin.

The actions of ice are:

restricts or completely stops bleeding
relieves pain after injury
numbs and desensitizes
protects body from overheating
checks all types of congestion
prevents swelling

eliminates fatigue
relieves joint pain
decongests head area
relieves depression
enhances memory

Often after strenuous physical work or engaging in sports, limbs and joints are stiff and their range of motion is limited. Ice restores to the joints a greater flexibility and mobility. Further, when ice is applied to the skin, it has a direct action on the nerve endings, making them less

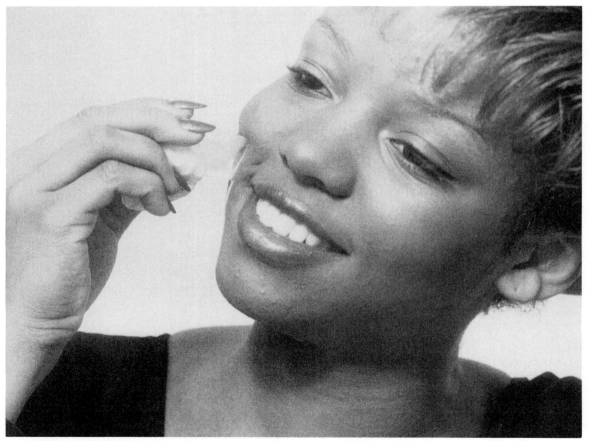

Ice will help tighten and tone sagging facial muscles. Hold an ice cube on your skin for fifteen seconds and remove. Repeat at least five times.

sensitive. Placing ice on wrists and other joints will help alleviate arthritic pain and swelling. Aches and pains will not be felt as readily with ice treatments. Is is usually best to apply ice directly and immediately to injuries to reduce edema (swelling due to water retention).

Another common use for ice is in reducing or preventing swelling. Since the cold temperature decreases the amount of pressure in the capillary vessels and lowers the extent of bleeding into the tissue spaces, swelling is reduced or completely inhibited. This is a partial explanation for the application of ice when there is a nosebleed. Cold temperatures act as vasoconstrictors as they inhibit blood flow. On the other hand, hot temperatures act as vasodilators as they increase blood flow; therefore one should never put anything warm or hot on the nose during a nosebleed.

For a nosebleed, hold ice (wrapped in a hand towel or cotton cloth, never directly on the skin) on one side of the nose and apply light pressure. Repeat this on the other side of the nose. If you feel the sense of tingling on the skin, remove for a minute or two. Usually you will find that holding the ice on for periods of thirty seconds at a time will be sufficient. Repeat the procedure until the bleeding has stopped.

Since the normal tendency of ice is to contract blood vessels, it relieves pressure from the entire circulatory system and the heart. When this happens, those who have hypertension experience a pleasant result: lowered blood pressure. The metabolic rate also decreases temporarily. Since the entire system slows down, the body has a chance to normalize and stabilize itself. In addition, ice decreases the inflammatory response and the production of tissue fluid, which results in a temporary weight loss.

There are a number of ways to apply ice:

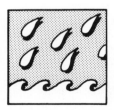

ICE PACKS

An ice pack consists of ice wrapped in a cloth or towel. It is used mainly to relieve pain and reduce swelling of the neck, joints, chest, head and back. To prepare an ice pack, it is easiest to use crushed ice. Depending on the size of the area you need to cover, crush a desired amount of ice and place it between a folded towel or cloth. Tie or wrap the towel or cloth in order to trap the cold. Hold the pack on the area involved. When you feel your skin throbbing, it is time to remove the pack so you do not damage the tissues. Short applications with the ice pack act as a tonic, while long applications lower temperature, lessen vital activity, as well as the body's production of heat. Add more ice to the cloth or towel when it begins to cool or melt.

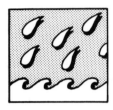 ## *ICE BAGS*

The ice bag is a waterproof rubber bag used for holding ice or extremely cold water. It is one of the most widely used forms of ice treatment, as it can be used as an ice pack but it has other uses as well. To use it, crush ice in large pieces and place them in the bag. Use a cloth or cotton towel between the ice bag and your skin. Apply the ice bag periodically, not continuously. Leave it on for a few minutes, take it off, then replace it, etc. The total time for an ice session should never exceed twenty to thirty minutes. If you need to hold the ice bag on for longer periods, it is possible to hold it in place with an elastic bandage, applying pressure to it. This will create a compress effect, enhancing its value. Another valuable technique to use in conjunction with the ice treatment is elevation. Elevation of a body part allows the blood to flow quickly in the direction of that part, thus bringing healing nutrients to the area.

77.2% of the earth's water is stored in the polar ice caps and glaciers. The largest body of frozen water is the Antarctic ice cap. It is more than 6,000,000 square miles. If it melts, it could fill the Mississippi River for more than 50,000 years.

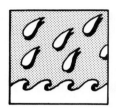

ICE-WATER IMMERSION

Ice immersion is a simple and natural water therapy. Many hospitals today are beginning to use ice immersion to treat chronic rheumatism, arthritis and kidney problems. It is a marvel of nature that allows us to

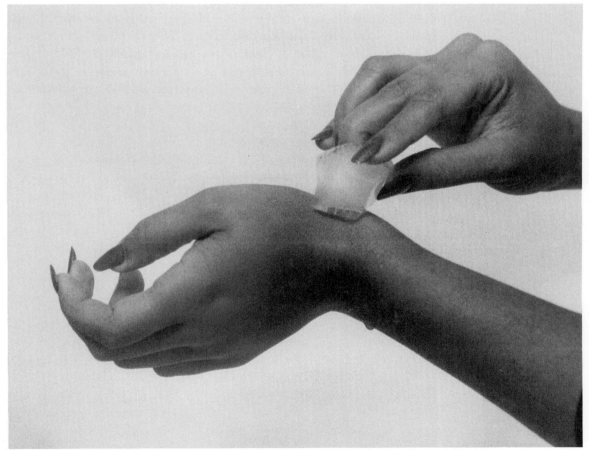

The properties of ice can make it both healing and regenerating. You may use it on any joint to increase circulation. Try it—it works!

positively affect the internal organs. Patients are subjected to periodic immersion in near-freezing water, staying in for up to five minutes. Shorter durations can also be effective.

There is a group called the Polar Bear Club whose members enjoy the ice-cold ocean by swimming in freezing waters in the winter. Their belief in the powers of cold water is so strong it enables them to create a frame of mind that allows the body to tolerate the otherwise dangerous temperatures. Members find the cold plunges revitalizing to the entire system.

If you are not quite ready for a Polar Bear plunge but still want an instant energy boost for your entire body, prepare a tub or pan of ice-cold water. Place your feet in the water and keep them in for at least thirty seconds. Take them out for one minute. Then, repeat the immersion for another thirty seconds. Repeat the entire procedure four or five times. At the end of the session, rinse your feet in warm water. You should feel refreshed and invigorated, no matter how tired you felt at the beginning.

11 HOT SPRINGS AND NATURAL SPAS

Water goes through a broad cycle in nature, passing around and through the earth. As rain, it falls to the earth, often sinking below the soil's surface, passes through mountains, travels along rock strata and eventually finds it way again to the surface. Along the way, it picks up minerals that become a part of its makeup. In many cases, these minerals provide the therapeutic qualities of spring water. In addition, air and sunshine contribute to water's potent power. Some water is held in rocks. The water is warmed because of being trapped between rocks that produce heat when they move and also because of volcanic action. Hot springs generally have a temperature between 96° and 110°F.

Sea water is another source of healing. Loaded with minerals, it, too, is used throughout the world for its special rejuvenating properties. The results can be long-term, or they can be immediate.

Thalassotherapy (*thalassa* is the Greek word for "sea") uses sea water and sea plants for both beauty and health purposes. A French biology professor named René Quinton found that plasma (the liquid part of blood) has a mineral content similar to that of sea water. The concept of thalassotherapy is based on the fact that the body absorbs sea water through the skin. The entire body, or only part of it, is wrapped in a sea plant, massaged and then sponged. The wrap is often warmed to add to its good feeling. The actions of mineral springs or sea water may benefit:

arthritis

poor circulation

nervous tension

sexual impotence

acne

chronic rheumatism

cellulite

burnout and depression

fatigue

muscle cramps and stiffness

There are healthy mineral waters on every continent of the earth, many of them with a history dating back centuries. Bathing in warm mineral springs is both enjoyable and healing. Much of this water is suitable for drinking and may also have a cleansing effect on the body. Trace elements are absorbed through the skin while showering or bathing in it, and many of these elements are important to the human body. Psychologically, troubles seem to melt away with a soak in a warm spring. As people pack their bodies with mud or seaweed, or plunge themselves into these waters, many hope the water lives up to its reputation as a healing force to rid their bodies of all ills.

History gives evidence of a spiritual connection between hot springs and human beings. Many ancient tales tell of friendly water spirits that keep watch over people and enliven them with special powers. Often religious celebrations or ceremonies took place around or near hot springs. Many Greek springs were, in fact, dedicated to the god Hercules, whose likeness can be found on coins excavated at the sites of the ancient spas.

Spas are as old as recorded history. In ancient Egypt, the builder Imotep constructed mineral-water houses in which the rich took rejuvenation baths. After coming out of the water, bathers then went to a special room where mud packs were applied and where they received full-body massages.

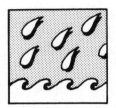

MINERAL BATHS

Mineral baths exist in a natural state all over the world. Their powers have been acclaimed throughout history and described as immediate. While recently speaking with a gentleman at my health club, I was

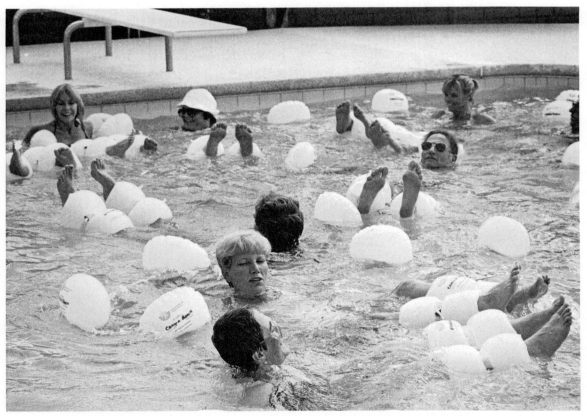

Water is now used by many people to enhance their overall health and is recommended by physical therapists and health maintenance counselors. Above, the happy gathering is enjoying the water while strengthening and toning muscles in the pool. *Photo courtesy of Canyon Ranch.*

thrilled to hear of his personal experiences with mineral waters. As it turned out, he owns a vast piece of property near Naples, Italy, on which four separate bodies of water exist. He described his experiences with one, a bubbling hot spring that has cured the aches and pains of his family for years. Another, a cold rush of water that is piped from a mountainside, is used by family and neighbors for all kinds of stomach and digestive problems. A third source is a warm spring that, he said, does everything from healing large cuts to clearing chronic skin problems.

Mineral baths are available at most spas and health resorts, and can be warm, hot, cool or cold. They are the oldest and most popular kind of therapeutic baths. It is essential to natural healing that they be preserved in their cleanest and most health-giving state, wherever they exist in the world. In ancient Rome there were over one thousand bathhouses or spas, using over 200 million gallons of water daily.

At the earliest spas, only massage, exercise and pleasure therapy (dance, theater and music) were offered to support the hydrotherapy treatments. People went there for weight loss, entertainment, social gossip, relaxation and beauty treatments. It was not long before a new enthusiasm for spas began to spread throughout the world. In Germany, whole towns were devoted to health spas; many of the towns can be

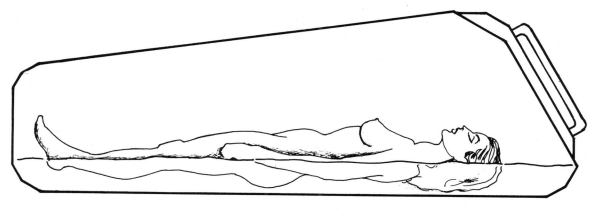

Flotation tanks are used by some therapists to offer their clients a state of total muscular and emotional relaxation. The client rests in a saline solution (essentially very salty water) in a completely unstimulated environment. The saline solution renders the body weightless and gravity-free.

identified by the word *Bad* (bath, bathhouse, spa) in their names. The wealthy began building luxurious villas near springs and lakes. For the last few centuries, the spa remained either a luxurious retreat for the wealthy or a pure health facility. Today, however, there is a new boom in the health spa, and it is patronized by people from all walks of life.

Modern spas fall into three general categories. The first group might be called the resort getaways. This type of facility, often described as a playground for the rich and famous, offers a complete selection of services. Its main characteristic is that the services are exclusive and usually expensive. If you can afford it, the price is usually well worth it. Catering to your every wish, resort getaways are the ultimate in healthy vacations. While their menus may contain healthy food, the presentations are usually gourmet feasts for your eyes. The approach stresses health blended with luxury.

The second type of spa is at the opposite end of the scale. The medical spa is primarily geared to treatment, through nonchemical means. Its main distinction is an in-depth, total approach to health. Along with a physician, nurses and technicians of many kinds help administer health and well-being programs. While such spas may be basic or luxurious, their environment is geared more to the physical care and rehabilitation of the body than to pleasureable distractions.

The third type of spa is the retreat. Retreats are temporary gatherings, workshops or group experiences held in temporary or permanent facilities, with or without luxurious and scenic environments. Juice fasts and special dieting or cleansing programs are often offered. Retreats may be held in or near the mountains or seaside, with all the comforts of a resort getaway. In addition, they can last any period of time, from one day to several months. Often, the retreat coordinators will arrange transportation and accommodations in advance for participants. Sponsors frequently conduct workshops and lectures (at which attendance is optional) on physical fitness and emotional and spiritual well-being. With more and more people in the workplace than ever, retreats also hold seminars on career development, personal motivation, stress management and other helpful subjects.

All three types of spas have their own special "something" that makes them unique. There are even spas that have combined the best features from all three types. Assess your needs and choose accordingly.

The features listed here will help you to decide on the kind of spa you are looking for:

1. mineral bath
2. sauna
3. steam bath
4. salt glow bath
5. herbal or mineral wrap
6. swimming pool
7. flotation tank
8. whirlpool
9. hot tub
10. mineral shower
11. massage
12. facial pack
13. exercise, equipment (Nautilus or free weights)
14. manicure, pedicure
15. solarium
16. archery
17. golf
18. dancing
19. medical evaluation
20. anti-stress program
21. weight-loss program
22. nutritional diet and counseling
23. aromatherapy
24. seminars, classes

In selecting a spa, there are several factors to consider in making it the best experience possible. Ask yourself what area you would like to be in. The physical location is one of personal choice. During the summer months, you might choose one location, and during the winter months, another climate and terrain may please you. Do you want to travel within the country, or outside of it? Would you prefer to be in the country, by the water or in the mountains? Why do you want to go? What is your purpose? What is the price of the stay, and which services are not included in the original cost? Which ones have extra fees? The prices at mineral springs tend to be reasonably fixed. The entrance fee will usually cover the use of natural mineral springs or a mineral water pool and even a massage or a mud bath. What is the general style? Is the atmosphere relaxed or formal and luxurious? Does it make you comfortable? What kind of food is served? Does your room have a view? Is it conveniently located? After you've answered these important questions, consider the programs at the various spas to find the one best suited to your needs.

Here are a few suggestions to consider.

Arizona—CANYON RANCH: Canyon Ranch offers you the opportunity to learn how to take charge of yourself, inside and out, as you relax and rejuvenate. The focus is on nutrition, fitness and stress management. It houses a 42,000-square-foot spa facility, featuring five gyms, a weight room, four racquetball courts and men's and women's quarters with steam rooms, saunas, Jacuzzis, inhalation therapy rooms, whirlpool baths, and areas for massage as well as beauty and skin care, and an historic clubhouse, with high-beamed ceilings. Open year-round.

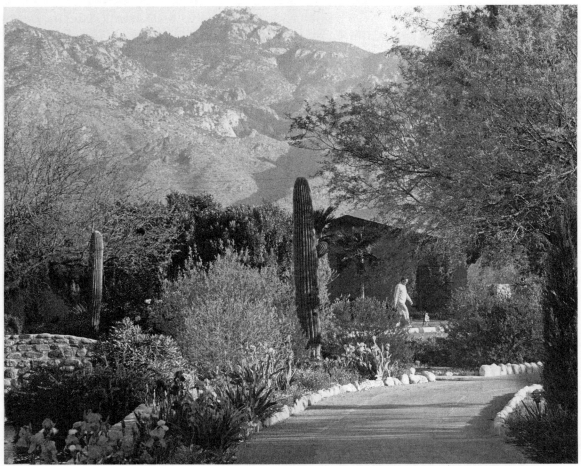

Today many resorts offer water therapies. Shown here is Canyon Ranch in Tucson, Arizona.

Arkansas—HOT SPRINGS: Hot Springs National Park is located in Arkansas, about fifty miles from Little Rock. It houses a number of bathhouses, and is adjacent to the National Park in the area. Open year-round.

California—GLEN IVY SPRINGS: The climate here is usually sunny. It is located two hours outside of Los Angeles in a pleasant desert setting. Water is of the mineral type and the springs are warm. Also offered are clay mudbaths. Open year-round.

Canada—JASPER NATIONAL PARK: Located in the Canadian Rockies, the setting is extremely beautiful and natural. The park has constructed a large public swimming pool to accommodate its many visitors. Open from May through August.

New Mexico—OJO-CALIENTE: The water here is hot and heavy, offering highly therapeutic benefits. Open year-round.

Virginia—WARM SPRINGS: Located about a five-hour drive from Washington, D.C., this is one of the oldest hot springs, in operation since 1761. Thomas Jefferson and James Madison went to Warm Springs for relaxation and health. The water is light and nearly five feet deep. Closed during the winter months.

Wyoming—YELLOWSTONE NATIONAL PARK: Also known as Boiling River, the park boasts a magnificent natural setting and lies near the Mammouth Hot Springs Hotel. The park's thermal mineral water reaches temperatures of 100°F and provides a unique healing property as it pours directly into the cold, fast-rushing Yellowstone River. Open year-round; free admission.

12

HOW TO FIX IT WITH WATER

The knowledge we have gained as to the therapeutic value of water can play a major role in our attempts to provide self-help care in both the prevention and relief of pain, discomfort or chronic problems. Water can be applied in specific ways to prevent and offer relief from many common stresses in our everyday lives. It can save us from making costly trips to and from the doctor's office or the local pharmacy. This is not to say that water in and of itself is a cure-all. But together with exercise, herbal plants, natural foods and mental well-being it can work harmoniously to offer a nontoxic program of stress reduction with little or no harmful side effects. That is one of the beauties of the natural way: There is the benefit of it working for us and very little chance that it will do us harm.

When applying water therapies, however, a little common sense should also be applied. Never overdo a treatment. When something is done in excess it is as bad as not doing it at all. Too much is as useless as too little. This applies especially to the temperature and duration of water applications. Try not to make your body uncomfortable with applications that are too hot or too cold.

Overall, you will find a world of both pleasure and therapeutic value in the discovery of water treatments. Welcome them with an open mind. Instead of reaching for the aspirin bottle during your next headache, try a warm relaxing compress instead. It just might work! Or try water treatments for any of the common ailments discussed below.

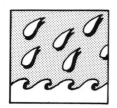

ABDOMINAL CRAMPS

Abdominal cramps are involuntary muscle contractions in the lower stomach and waist area. These contractions can cause pain and discomfort. For relief, try the following water therapies:

- Apply a warm pack on the abdominal area for fifteen minutes. If the pack cools during that period, exchange it for a warmer one.
- Apply a hot, moist compress to the stomach and back (it must be large enough to fit this area). Wrap it around your waist and clip or tie it in the front. Leave the compress on for at least ten minutes.
- Take a warm bath, sitting in water up to your waist.
- Drink a cup of warm peppermint or camomile tea.

Deep, slow breathing may also be useful to relieve cramps and tightness and tension in the stomach area. Or try massaging warm oil (peppermint or olive) into the stomach area in small, light, circular motions. Massage clockwise first, then counterclockwise, alternating every few minutes.

Please note that severe or persistent abdominal pain should always be discussed with a physician. Major causes of abdominal discomfort include fear, anxiety, eating the wrong foods and weak stomach or back muscles.

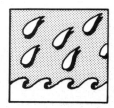

ARTHRITIS

Arthritis is characterized by inflammation and pain in the joints. All forms of arthritis respond well to water treatments. Here are some hints for relief:

1. Drink plenty of fresh pure water. Distilled water can be beneficial as a cleanser that absorbs acid.
2. Take alternating hot and cold showers. Start with fifteen minutes of hot water, then switch to five minutes of cool water. Apply the shower spray directly to the wrist, ankle or other specific part.
3. Water exercises in the tub or pool can soothe minor discomfort. For the wrist or ankle, place either underwater. Push the water gently back and forth with your hand or foot. Range-of-motion rotations may also be used.
4. Leave a cotton or wool glove in the freezer for ten minutes or more. When it is as cold as you can stand it, pull it out. Quickly wash your hands in hot/warm water. Put the cold glove on immediately and leave it on for about ten minutes. Remove the glove, wash your hands in neutral water and massage them with olive oil for fifteen minutes. Massage them daily for fifteen minutes.
5. Mustard packs (see page 118 for instructions on making a mustard pack) or sage packs will soothe arthritic inflammation.
6. Swimming increases the mobility of stiff joints.
7. Sage, rosemary, camomile, and comfrey teas have a therapeutic value in arthritis.

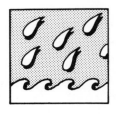

LOWER BACK PAIN

The lower back is involved in 70 percent of all human movement. Therefore, its muscles are prone to excessive stress and exertion. Weak stomach muscles, improper lifting, kidney problems and worry are just a few of the causes of lower back pain. People who exhibit poor posture, wear high heels too frequently and sit too long often experience lower back pain.

Swimming is the best exercise for the lower back. If you must work sitting, find a pillow that supports and takes the strain from your back.

Be aware of your posture, as slumping and drooping in your chair will cause a strain on your back. There are, however, many other practical remedies for lower back pain:

1. *Exercise*—Lie flat on your stomach, inhale and lift your legs at the waist. Hold your feet off the ground about twelve inches, for a count of ten. Lower them slowly. After repeating this three times, lift your knees to your chest, clasping your hands around your knees. Rock back and forth on your buttocks and lower back. Breathe in and out slowly. Try to visualize the tension flowing out of your back area and disappearing in the air around you.

2. *Hot packs*—These work wonders when you place them on your lower back. Lie flat on your stomach. Make sure the pack is as warm as you can stand it. Place the pack over your lower back. Begin to breathe deeply, inhaling and exhaling. As you exhale, use the visualization technique to expel the tension from the area. Take your time, and relax. When you relax totally, your muscles will work in support of your actions and not against them.

3. *Massage*—Using a cotton towel, place it around your waist and hold on to the ends. Move the towel back and forth, massaging the muscles in your lower back.

For long-term relief and prevention of lower back pain, it is imperative to strengthen stomach and back muscles.

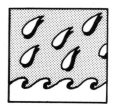 ## *STRESS AND ANXIETY*

Put simply, stress and anxiety are a result of too many of the wrong things too often. If you are experiencing undue stress and strain, change your habits. Replace old health-threatening life patterns with fresh, new, health-supporting ones. This will require you first to identify the emotional, physical, nutritional and social aspects of your life that are creating disharmony in your current life. Once you begin to tackle those areas, keep in mind these water techniques that will aid you in relieving and preventing stress and anxiety:

1. First—again—is swimming. It is the single best way to relax, tone and invigorate your body.
2. The whirlpool and hot tub offer a place for you to get away from it all, while the heat and whirling water soothe your tight, tense muscles.
3. Cold packs to the head will help focus your mind and slow it down when it begins to race and get out of control.
4. Drinking plenty of fresh spring water, along with reducing your intake of sugar and fried foods and cessation of smoking, will bring harmony to your body.
5. There are herbal teas that seem to have a direct connection with the body's ability to relax. They include: camomile, valerian, hops and jasmine. All can be purchased from a health-food store and easily made into a calming drink, mixed with pure honey.

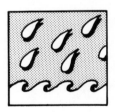 ## *INTERNAL IMPURITIES*

Constipation and indigestion are at the root of many imbalances. Since the elimination system plays a major role in good health, internal cleansing is a superior way to guarantee your body stays at an optimal level of fitness. To clean the entire system, do the following:

1. Drink as much pure natural water as possible.
2. Ask your physician about colonics (high enemas). Have one at least once a year, if not more. Herbal teas that cleanse the internal body include: peppermint, comfrey, alfalfa, dandelion, cascara sagrada (an excellent bowel cleanser) and psyllium. (Psyllium is a small seed that expands into a bulk material when

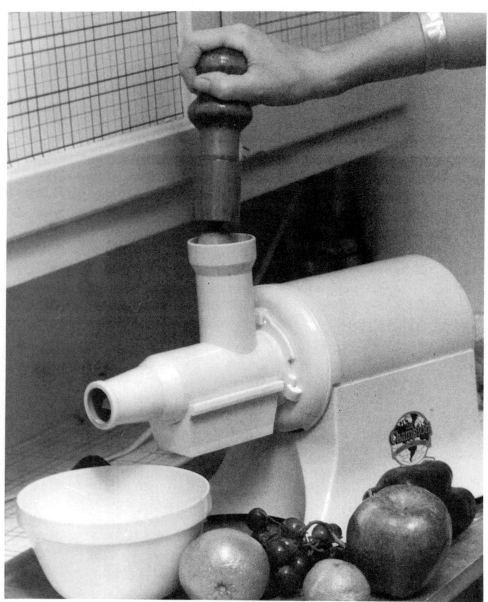

Most fruits and vegetables—like the human body—are composed largely of water. In addition, they are filled with vitamins, minerals and life-giving enzymes. Juicers extract these natural properties easily and should be part of your health and beauty program.

it is mixed with water. Many pharmaceuticals use it in laxative formulas. It, too, can be purchased from a health-food store. It may be mixed with bentonite, green clay, and sold as an internal cleanser. The psyllium is used to cleanse the colon, the bentonite to purify the blood.)

3. Take a relaxing swim, regularly. Stress, worry, fear and anger create impurities in your body, especially the liver, which functions as the body's filtering system.

4. Apply hot compresses to the abdomen; they will aid your stomach when it is upset. After the hot compress, massage your abdomen in small, circular motions for ten minutes. This will help to improve elimination.

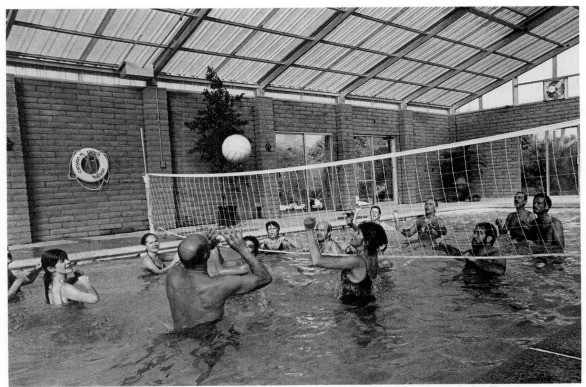

Water sports fun: These people are enjoying the pool at Canyon Ranch in Tucson, Arizona, while toning and strengthening all their muscles. *Photo courtesy of Canyon Ranch.*

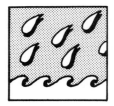

CELLULITE

While it won't prevent cellulite from forming (cellulite occurs when fluid and fat are trapped together below the skin and form pockets, especially around hips, thighs and stomach), hydrotherapy *will* help reduce its unsightly appearance:

1. Wet-brush massage is used in some spas to stimulate the circulation and dissolve some of the trapped pockets. Use a loofah or soft natural bristle brush and massage vigorously, in circular motions. This should be done for about five minutes at a time. After the circular motions, rub a small amount of olive oil into the area, and grasp the area between your four fingers and thumb and knead it deeply.
2. Drink plenty of fresh spring water.
3. Adding a tablespoon of apple cider vinegar to your water in the morning will help dissolve cellulite.
4. Leg exercises in the tub or pool will tighten thighs and hips.

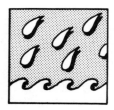

HEADACHE

There are a number of different types of headaches. They all share one thing in common—discomfort. Often a good night's sleep, exercise and fresh air will calm and soothe the nervous system and ease the discomfort associated with a headache. For immediate relief, try the following hydrotherapy techniques:

1. Apply a warm compress to the special headache reflex point located in the center rear of your neck; use gentle pressure.

2. Soak your feet in warm water. A foot soak may be one of the best and oldest remedies for a headache. It relieves pressure on the head by attracting circulation to the feet and lower extremities.

3. Draw a warm bath, lie back and relax. Perform eight to ten neck rotations in each direction. Then, use a relaxing visualization in which you see the tension release itself and float out of your head area, dissipating into the air. (Deep breathing is also excellent for calming the body, since headaches are usually accompanied by stressful thoughts pounding away inside our heads.)

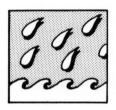

BURNOUT

As the world becomes a more active place, with louder noises, increased use of pesticides and an overall accelerated pace, the human body has remained the same. How do we cope with these uncontrolled changes around us? How do we maintain optimal health and fitness, and at the same time enjoy the many fruits and pleasures life has to offer? Maintaining a proper balance between the two is the answer.

Water, because of its cost-effectiveness, accessibility and practicality, will help serve this purpose. Its qualities are rejuvenating and invigorating. Water stimulates, energizes and helps us maintain an optimal level of fitness. What is even better is that it carries with it very few harmful side effects and is almost impossible to abuse. To counteract the exhaustion that comes with burnout, try the following water therapies:

1. Start with a cold bath. It will rejuvenate frazzled nerves and begin the invigorating mechanism. Or, for a time-saving device, try a cold shower.

2. Cold compresses to the head and cold foot baths at the same time are wonderful for getting the juices flowing.

3. Swimming at least three times a week is perhaps the best all-around energizer.

4. Drink plenty of fresh water.

Finally, a word of advice: Don't worry, take life in stride, enjoy and live life to its fullest. Put more of the simple things in life into your activities—they are usually best. Get lots of sunshine, breathe fresh air, eat healthful foods and think positive thoughts.

THE AUNU BEAUTY LINE

The Aunu Beauty Line is a collection of easy-to-use products that help renew the skin at a deep cellular level. It should be part of a health and beauty program for every active, health-conscious person today.

Geared for the personal skin-care needs of all ages and most skin types, these fine products are hypoallergenic and contain only the finest natural ingredients available. Scientifically tested, they have been mixed to adjust to your skin chemistry for the correct pH factor.

Aunu Moisture Creme

A super moisture-retaining product, Aunu Moisture Creme nourishes your skin and acts to decelerate the aging process by diminishing unwanted wrinkles. Hypoallergenic and dermatologist-recommended, the creme contains the complete group of amino-acid concentrates combined with the nourishing properties of aloe vera, bee pollen, camomile, vitamin E, collagen and elastin to penetrate deep into your underlying cellular tissue to restore skin elasticity, aid in cell regeneration and create a new life for your skin.

Aunu Herbal Sauna

A safe, easy method of deep-cleaning your pores and stimulating your skin for a healthier complexion. Treat yourself to a warm, aromatic vapor that will open blocked sinuses and nasal passages while also relaxing facial muscles. Blended from a liquid potpourri of fresh peppermint, purified water, eucalyptus, lavender, comfrey, camomile and pure peach oil, the Aunu Herbal Sauna will leave your skin clean and baby-soft.

For more information, or to order Aunu products, write to Aunu Cosmetics, Box 18613, Washington, DC 20036. Be sure to enclose your name and address with your inquiry.

13 DRINKING WATER

The demand for clean drinking water has increased dramatically during this decade, primarily because most of our tap water is outright polluted and contains chemicals that are toxic. As a result, there are now over 450 bottling plants in the United States alone. They produce more than 600 different brands of water. Over 50 brands of imported waters are also available, most of them naturally carbonated mineral waters.

There are several types of drinking waters, depending on the source of the water. How do you know when you are getting pure water? What are the differences between the various classifications of water?

Drinking water is bottled water obtained from an approved source. It has undergone special treatment, or has undergone a minimum treatment, consisting of filtration and ozonation or an equivalent disinfection process.

Natural water is bottled spring, mineral, artesian well or well water derived from an underground formation, not from a municipal system of public water supply. It is unmodified by blending with water from another source, or by the addition or deletion of dissolved solids, except as it relates to ozonation or equivalent disinfection and filtration.

Spring water is derived from an underground formation from which water flows naturally to the surface of the earth. Spring water should also meet the requirements of natural water.

Well water is bottled water from a hole bored, drilled or otherwise constructed in the ground, which taps the water of an aquifer.

Distilled (purified) water is bottled water produced by distillation, deionization or reverse osmosis. Water that is vaporized and then condensed can be labeled distilled (or purified) water. Only water prepared by distillation can be labeled distilled water.

When purchasing purified bottled water, remember that some are merely reconstituted distilled or deionized tap water and that plastic bottles sometimes leak their petrochemicals into the water.

In the distillation process, water is vaporized and then condensed, leaving behind dissolved minerals. In deionization, water is passed through resins that remove most of the dissolved minerals. Reverse osmosis involves forcing water under pressure through membranes that remove 90 percent of dissolved minerals.

Club sodas and seltzer waters are generally used as mixes or sodas, or as soft drinks. They contain artificial carbonation. Minerals are added to club soda but not to seltzer; otherwise they are the same.

The Food and Drug Administration, which regulates bottled water as a food, has declined to define mineral water or natural water. Several states have regulations requiring a water to contain not less than 500 parts per million total dissolved solids in order to be labeled a mineral water. The International Bottled Water Association, the trade association for the bottled-water industry, has adopted the following definitions:

Mineral water—bottled water is defined as water that contains not less than 500 parts per million total dissolved solids. *Carbonated or sparkling water*—naturally carbonated mineral water or naturally sparkling mineral water is defined as water whose carbon dioxide content is from the same source as the water; carbonated natural water or sparkling natural water is defined as water to which has been added carbon dioxide of an origin other than the deposit from which the water comes; carbonated drinking water is defined as water to which has been added carbon dioxide of an origin other than the source water.

Distilled water contains nothing but hydrogen and oxygen. It is pure water; however, because the minerals and other organic substances have been removed, it is not wise to drink it for prolonged periods of time. It is, however, superior in fasts and cleansings of all types since it absorbs toxins and impurities for elimination.

Bottled water is free of chlorine, as the final purifying agent used by most bottled water companies is O_3, a form of oxygen. Unlike chlorine, which is commonly used by public water supplies, ozone leaves no residual aftertaste or smell.

Domestic water is regulated by the federal government and by all state and some local agencies. All bottled water is bottled under strict sanitary conditions. The International Bottled Water Association, founded in 1958, represents over 90 percent of the total company sales in the U.S. The association also has international bottlers who both sell and distribute imported waters in the U.S. (For further information, contact them at 113 North Henry Street, Alexandria, Virginia; 703- 683-5213.)

Selection of bottled water is strictly a matter of personal preference. All waters are classified by their taste as well as their content. The next time you want to have some fun, have a water-tasting session. Once you

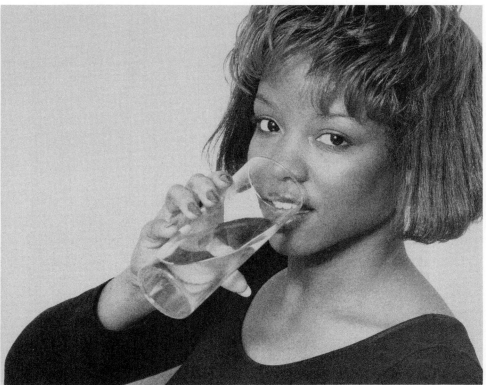

Just a good glass of fresh, pure drinking water!

get turned on to the gourmet aspect of water, you will have opened up an entirely new world of pleasure.

Rate the various brands on taste, mineral content and availability. You will notice that some are clear, with almost no taste, some are bubbly, others are not. Some have a pleasing medicinal taste, while others are flat. Here's a partial list of brands:

Apollinaris—somewhat salty
Canada Dry—strong carbonation
Perrier—mildly carbonated
Poland Spring—pure neutral taste, carbonated
Ramlösa—mild mineral flavor
San Pellegrino—slightly tart, lightly carbonated
Saratoga—medium tart, very slight mineral taste
Evian—pure taste
Mountain Valley—pure, healthy taste

Water is a natural healer as well as a thirst-quencher. The actions of drinking water are:

bathes internal organs
stimulates kidney function
helps respiration
regulates body temperature
rejuvenates all cells
activates digestive and eliminative organs
provides a source of energy and nourishment
dilutes body fluids
eliminates toxins
helps relieve arthritis
promotes moist, supple skin
purifies blood

So, whether you choose tap water or one of the waters just described, drink up!

14
A WET FUTURE

We live in a fast-paced, high-tech world. Where there is high technology and high industry, there are bound to be residual chemicals and pollutants of all types that fill the water supply. The waste materials dumped in our water is enormous. A recent survey of public water systems, served by ground water, showed 55 percent of them to be polluted at dangerous levels by organic chemicals. According to a survey by the Environmental Protection Agency, two-thirds of the nation's households were drinking water that does not meet all of its health standards. Americans now spend over 2.5 billion dollars a year on bottled water and home filters to combat this problem.

The Environmental Protection Agency was designed by Congress to set nationwide standards and back them up by imposing stiff financial penalties. About one in four Americans develops cancer; some 20 percent of American couples cannot conceive, and a large percentage of pregnancies end in miscarriage. Contaminated water may be one of the main culprits.

Chemical contamination of our water supply has become the most serious environmental problem of our time. Most troublesome is pollution affecting our ground water. Streams, rivers and lakes hold only about 4 percent of the water in the U.S. The rest lies from three feet to hundreds of feet below the surface, unseen in vast reservoirs called aquifers. In places like California and New Jersey, the water supply of nearly every underground aquifer is polluted.

Ground water is not isolated from surface water. The two are intimately connected. Ground water outcrops into springs and contributes about 30 percent of the volume of the nation's streams, lakes and rivers.

Rain and surface waters, in turn, seep down through the earth to replenish ground water. Ground water provides drinking water for half the population of the U.S. and more than 90 percent of rural residents.

Our use of ground water has tripled since 1950 and indications are that it will be our main source of fresh water in the future. Many industrial and agricultural chemicals have found their way into ground water. Chemicals from hazardous waste sites; heavy metals and radioactive substances from mining; gasoline from underground storage tanks; pesticides and nitrates used in agriculture; salt from road de-icing; bacteria from leaky septic tanks—all are sources of pollutants.

In 1974, the EPA announced that its tests identified no less than sixty-six different organic chemicals in the drinking water of New Orleans. Congress passed a Safe Drinking Water Act, which gave the EPA the power to set and enforce safe exposure levels for toxic substances in drinking water. Thousands of tons of chemical wastes in landfills, dumps, pits and ponds were slowly seeping through the ground into the underlying water table. Once there, they would then make their way toward nearby drinking water wells.

Reports have linked toxic chemicals in drinking water to cancer, birth defects, kidney and liver ailments, headaches, skin problems and mental disorders. Trichlorethylene, a clear, colorless liquid, is now widely used as a solvent and degreaser in industrial processes and in consumer products. In high doses, TCE can cause the above-mentioned health problems.

Because ground water stores chemicals that do not dissipate, in time, the toxic levels in ground water may increase as more chemical pollutants seep through the soil and enter the aquifers. A contaminant that penetrates ground water tends to form a layer of contaminated water moving slowly through the aquifer for years or decades and even longer.

After World War II, a virtual explosion of chemicals found their way into almost every type of industrial and consumer product imaginable. Synthetic fibers replaced natural ones; plastic replaced wood, glass and metal.

In 1988, it was estimated the U.S. was producing somewhere between 24 and 54 million tons of hazardous chemical wastes each year. It stands to reason that if chemicals are put into the ground, they will eventually end up in the water supply.

Thus far, most states dump brine into pits, where it eventually soaks into the ground and into the ground water. Each year, we put over 10 billion gallons of sewage into the earth. Gasoline may be responsible for as much as 40 percent of the nation's ground water contamination. The EPA estimates that up to a fourth of our 2.5 million gasoline storage tanks may be leaky. Near mines, water may contain arsenic, a heavy metal linked to cancer, nerve disorders and digestive tract disorders.

Equally tragic is the fact that millions of specimens of aquatic life are being poisoned and many die as a result. Acid drainage from coal

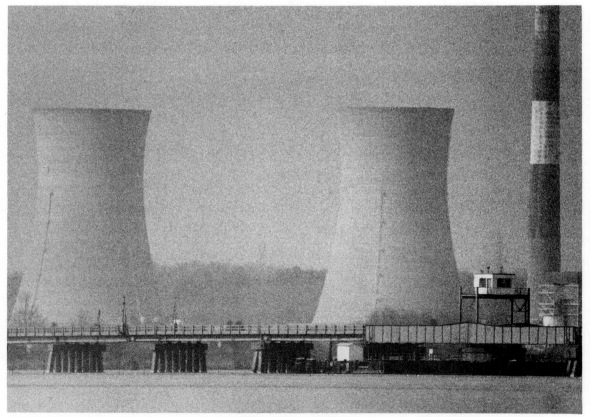

The future of our home water source depends upon the care we take of our environment. Above, city water supplies are held in large water tanks that, because of the sophisticated filtration devices involved, resemble nuclear power plants. *Photo by Steve Delaney/EPA.*

mines has caused severe water-quality problems in more than 3,000 miles of streams in Pennsylvania, West Virginia, Maryland and Virginia.

Nuclear plants release a massive amount of chemical waste. It is laced with deadly radioactivity, which can damage cells and lead to unhealthy conditions. The 27-square-mile Rocky Mountain Arsenal near Denver, Colorado, is laced with contaminated land and water. Over eight hundred wells in Florida are contaminated with EDB, Ethylene Dibromide, a toxic chemical which has also been found in the water in Hawaii, California, Virginia, Massachusetts, South Carolina, Washington State, Connecticut and Arizona. Pesticides have been found in

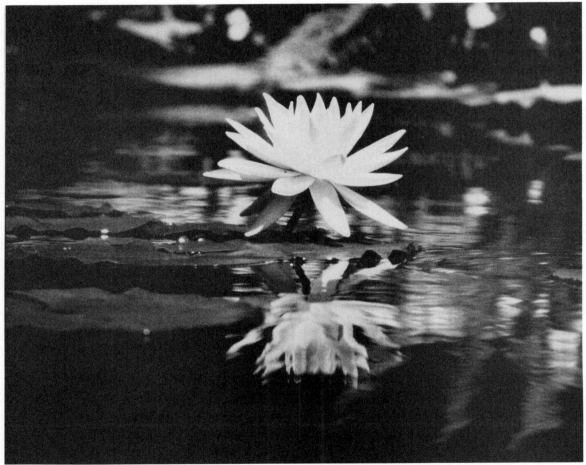

Water lilies: This type of flower lives on the water. *Photo © Lilyponds Water Gardens.*

ground water in more than twenty states. The main source of nitrates in ground water is nitrogen-based fertilizer that leaches through the soil into the water table. High levels of nitrates can cause oxygen depletion in infants.

The way we treat and transport our water may pose serious health problems in itself. We rely on a maze of underground pipelines totaling a million miles nationwide to deliver more than 30 billion gallons of water annually. There are over 50,000 public and private water companies in the U.S. Some cities obtain water from nearby rivers, while others pump water from up to 300 miles away. When water comes out of the tap, it has been transformed, passed through screens to keep out debris and fish and mechanically mixed with chemicals to destroy bad taste and odors. To kill bacteria it is run through a series of baffles to give the chemicals more time to act. It is then gathered in ponds to allow the sediment to settle out and then pumped under tremendous pressure to consumers.

Chlorine and filters are used to kill bacteria in water. Chlorine was first added in 1908, when a small amount of bleaching powder was added to a reservoir in New Jersey. Eventually, all public health officials began adding chlorine to finished drinking water. Chlorination in itself, however, may lead to carcinogenic contamination in the form of trihalomethanes.

Sixty percent of the American population now drinks artificially fluoridated water. Fluoride is a compound found in almost all soils, plants and water. In the United States, the belief is that fluoride, added to water in certain concentrates, reduces dental cavities. Some claim, however, that long-term exposure to fluoridated drinking water can weaken the immune system.

Plastic pipe used in household plumbing and solvent glues used to join sections of the pipe contain dimethylformamide, a chemical linked to birth defects. In addition, certain respiratory and lung conditions have been linked to their use. As water flows through plastic pipe, chemicals leak into the water, along with gasoline and other substances.

To combat these toxins, many companies now market home purification devices. Have your water tested first to determine exactly what type of purification system you need. There is no such thing as pure water—even the clearest untreated tap water contains mineral salts, trace metals and organic matter. Some of these substances are beneficial and others harmful. Often, the taste, color or smell may let you know that your water is unsafe. Brown stains left around your sink indicate high levels of iron, while green stains indicate elevated levels of copper. A metallic taste may indicate deteriorating pipes, chemical leakage from new plumbing, or other chemical contaminants. Radon gas, a naturally occurring radioactive substance, is found in ground water, and many areas have high levels of sulfur, calcium and uranium.

Water filters will remove only certain contaminants. Domestic devices that remove bacteria and viruses are technically known as purifiers.

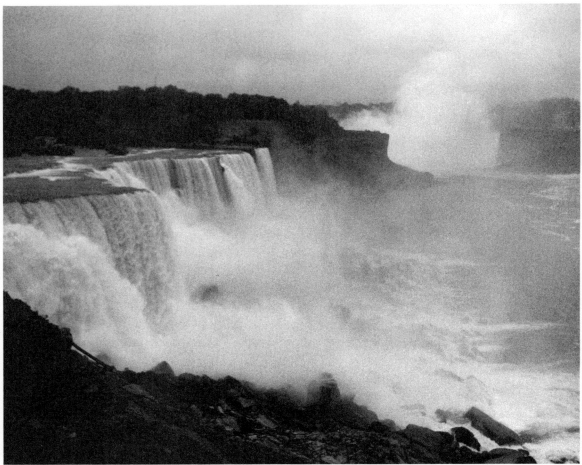

The first shower.

Any filter system that does not perform this function cannot be legally called a purifier. Water purifiers commonly employ a chemical feeder that injects small amounts of chlorine either into the well or into the water. Iodine is also an efficient disinfectant, but it is not considered safe for use by pregnant women.

Water softeners also change the chemical makeup of water. They remove calcium and magnesium ions, responsible for hard water, but the water produced by these appliances contains elevated levels of salt, which is linked with high blood pressure and hypertension.

Some municipal water systems use ultraviolet light to kill bacteria and to reduce organic chemicals. Water passes through clear glass tubes and is subjected to ultraviolet light and certain organic chemicals, and is altered in such a way that the chemicals and bacteria are not harmful. UV systems are ineffective if the water is slightly clouded, however. Bacteria actually cling to particles in the water and are protected from UV light. UV light also has difficulty penetrating anything that is not clear; clearing the glass tubes of scale and debris and replacing burned-out light bulbs correct this.

In UV home treatment units, which are still in the developmental stage, microorganisms are exposed to UV radiation from a lamp that shines on the water as it flows by. Their effectiveness is reduced in water with high turbidity or high iron levels.

Reverse osmosis systems are quickly becoming the standard in home water treatment devices. The process involves three filters, arranged in a series. Water from a cold water line first enters a sediment filter, which removes large particulate matter. Without this component, the system would soon be filled with sediment. The pore size of the membrane in the sediment filter is from one to five microns, or about the diameter of a human hair. The filter consists of a paper cartilage inside a plastic cannister. (Some units have clear plastic containers so you can see the amount of sediment that has been strained from the water.)

The water then enters a second cannister, containing the reverse osmosis membranes. These membranes resemble cellophane. The units work very slowly because the pore size is such that only a single water molecule can pass through at a time. Water is forced against an outer layer of the membrane. Here, the initial separation of contaminants from the water molecule occurs. The large contaminants are flushed from the membrane surface with waste water, and the smaller water molecules are squeezed through with ultrafine membrane pores. Each successive layer of membrane further refines the water so that clean water finally reaches a tub in the center, which is connected to the last filter cannister.

The third cannister contains an activated carbon filter cartridge, which removes contaminants, especially lighter-weight organic contaminants and dissolved gases that may have passed through the osmosis system.

Reverse osmosis systems are quiet and effective. The membrane cartridges must be replaced in time, carbon filters more often, and sediment filters are also necessary. The units depend on water pressure for proper operation. They will not perform if the pressure is below thirty-five pounds per square inch.

Activated carbon filters are sold through retail stores and can be found in a variety of designs. However, bacteria may breed in the carbon. The problem results from the carbon inside the filter. Smaller units contain too little activated carbon to be effective. Large filters are better and give longer service life. Activated carbon is highly porous—one pound of activated charcoal has a surface area of one acre. Molecules passing over the surface area are captured by the carbon. Activated carbon is available in three forms. Avoid powdered carbon since it is subject to release particles of carbon into the finished water; if particles are charged with contaminants, you will consume concentrated doses of the chemicals you intend to remove. Granulated charcoal is found in the majority of filters. The particles are larger. Water passes through the filter, in channels between the granules. Because this reduces the amount of carbon available to filtration, these filters should be equipped with a back flush valve to rearrange and clean the carbon. Solid block activated charcoal filters are considered superior. Channeling cannot occur and the solid block filters usually last longer, compensating for their higher cost.

Several types of filter are available. Sink-mounted models are placed on the end of the faucet. Most have a bypass so that you have the option of drawing unfiltered water for washing. Under-the-sink models are usually larger and use a cannister or cartridge connected with the cold water line. Most offer the option of allowing unfiltered water to be trapped separately. Pour-through and appliance units operate independently of the plumbing system. Much like a pour-through coffeemaker, water is poured through a filter cannister and into a vessel. Some units employ a small electric pump to force the water through the unit continuously to remove more contaminants with each passage through the carbon. Under-the-sink models are proven to be more effective than smaller, end-of-faucet models in removing undesirable materials. Carbon filters are not very effective at removing dissolved materials such as heavy metals from your water. They are also ineffective against most types of bacteria.

The filtration process used in home distillers is much like the solar-powered hydrological cycle in nature: When the heat of the sun turns water into vapor, solid impurities are left behind. The vapor condenses back into water particles as it is drawn into the atmosphere. These water particles appear as naturally distilled dew, rain or snow.

In a distiller, water is either poured or fed automatically into a vaporizing chamber, where it is then boiled by an electrical resistance heating element. As the steam rises, most chemicals, minerals, bacteria, viruses and other pollutants are removed. Distillers should be cleaned periodically to remove sediment that builds up over time.

By now it should be abundantly clear that we must do something to prevent further destruction of our waters, something to purify the water we have and something that helps create new sources from currently unavailable sources. The task is not impossible. It begins with taking better care of what water we already have. Water is a precious substance, vital in every part of our lives. Its flowing movement is graceful, its energy magnetic. Water is a substance so valuable that entire wars are fought over its ownership, a substance so stable that blocks of it have been frozen and remained solid in the same place, for eons.

Perhaps, if every single person cares, then together the unity of our loving efforts for the simple survival of pure, usable water will show positive results in the future.

Just think about it: What would *your* life be like without water?

Practicing the ancient art of divining.

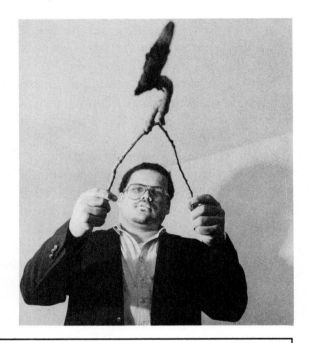

Finding Water with a Rod

The science of divining or dowsing is not all hocus-pocus. Bristol-Myers actually paid a diviner, or dowser (one who locates underground sources of water or minerals), to locate a water source for its plant in New Jersey. The diviner located an underground stream with water that flowed at 175 gallons per minute! RCA and DuPont are among the many other companies that have used diviners with success. Diviners have also been hired by home builders and well drillers.

A diviner uses a divining rod to locate water sources underground. Most diviners use a Y-shaped rod made of wood. The rod is held in front of the diviner, who keeps elbows out, fists tight and palms up on the two sides of the rod. If the rod moves dramatically, or moves up or down, there is the possibility that water is near. In the pendulum method, an object is dangled from a string or chain. If it swings or shakes, water is nearby.

Anyone can be trained to be a diviner, with the proper sensitivity. But, let's face it, some people were just made to search for and locate water sources through the oldest method known to mankind.